DAILY SEX
BIBLE

DAILY SEX BIBLE

INSPIRATIONS AND TECHNIQUES FOR THE BEST YEAR OF SEX EVER

SUSAN CRAIN BAKOS

Author of *The Sex Bible, The Sex Bible for Women,* and *The Orgasm Bible*

Text © 2010 Susan Crain Bakos
Photography © 2010 Quiver

First published in the USA in 2010 by
Quiver, a member of
Quayside Publishing Group
100 Cummings Center
Suite 406-L
Beverly, MA 01915-6101
www.quiverbooks.com

The Publisher maintains the records relating to images in this book required by 18
USC 2257. Records are located at Rockport Publishers, Inc., 100 Cummings Center,
Suite 406-L, Beverly, MA 01915-6101.

14 13 12 11 10 1 2 3 4 5

ISBN-13: 978-1-59233-447-6
ISBN-10: 1-59233-447-4

Library of Congress Cataloging-in-Publication Data available

Cover design by Carol Holtz
Book design by sporto
Photography by [Please enter]

Printed and bound in Singapore

Contents

WEEK 5 Devoted to the Study of the Classics	WEEK 6 Sexy Thighs and Discoveries	WEEK 7 Pursuing Sensual Delights	WEEK 8 Unexpected Pleasures	WEEK 9 The Forgotten Zones
Day 29: Seducing the Nipple **(52)**	**Day 36:** Thigh-High Kissing **(60)**	**Day 43:** Tantalizing the Taste Buds **(68)**	**Day 50:** Double Entendres and Coffee **(76)**	**Day 57:** Back-to-Back Snuggle **(84)**
Day 30: The Hand-Job Quickie, Hers **(53)**	**Day 37:** The Morning Quickie **(61)**	**Day 44:** Redefining "Sex" **(69)**	**Day 51:** The Naked Chef **(77)**	**Day 58:** The Vibe/Tongue/G-Spot Triple-Play Quickie, Hers **(84)**
Day 31: Historical BJ #1: Catherine The Great's Special **(54)**	**Day 38:** The Clitoral Roots, an Anatomy Lesson **(62)**	**Day 45:** The Corona Lick #1 **(70)**	**Day 52:** The "Cum Shake" **(79)**	**Day 59:** The Historical BJ #2: The Duchess of Windsor's Butterfly Throat **(85)**
Day 32: The A-Frame Effect **(55)**	**Day 39:** The New Woman on Top #1: The Shy Reverse Cowgirl **(63)**	**Day 46:** Her Multiple Os #1: Compounded Single Orgasms **(71)**	**Day 53:** The fMRI Orgasm **(80)**	**Day 60:** The Secret Orgasm Mind Set, Hers **(86)**
Day 33: Painting Her O **(56)**	**Day 40:** The Roman Romp **(65)**	**Day 47:** Her Striptease **(73)**	**Day 54:** Create a Toy Box **(81)**	**Day 61:** Anal Orgasm, His **(88)**
Day 34: Arab Sex #3: The Art of Brinksmanship **(57)**	**Day 41:** Questing for G-Spots: His and Hers **(66)**	**Day 48:** Arab Sex #4: Ejaculatory Control **(74)**	**Day 55:** The 2,000-Year-Old BJ Position **(82)**	**Day 62:** Puritan Sex: Repressed but Dirty#1, Clothes On **(89)**
Day 35: The Legend of the Lingam **(58)**	**Day 42:** A Pussy Altar **(67)**	**Day 49:** The Legend of the Yoni **(75)**	**Day 56:** Kundalini #1: Freeing the Energy **(83)**	**Day 63:** The Spiritual Orgasm #1: Extra-Genital **(90)**

WEEK 15 Light and Sexy	WEEK 16 Start Fast, End Slow	WEEK 17 The Poetry of Sexual Expansion	WEEK 18 Sexual Mind Shifts	WEEK 19 The Penis Pushes Up the Week
Day 99: New Lingerie Day **(132)**	**Day 106:** The Fast Hot(ter) Shower **(140)**	**Day 113:** Erotic Poetry **(148)**	**Day 120:** Spider Walk **(156)**	**Day 127:** Penis Push-Ups **(164)**
Day 100: The "Not-in-the-Mood" Quickie **(132)**	**Day 107:** The Mutual Masturbation with Sex Toys Quickie **(141)**	**Day 114:** The "Affair" Quickie **(149)**	**Day 121:** Mental Foreplay **(157)**	**Day 128:** The Light-His Fire Quickie **(165)**
Day 101: Tea-Bagging, His **(133)**	**Day 108:** The Rock 'n' Roll CJ, Hers **(142)**	**Day 115:** The Rock 'n' Roll BJ, His **(150)**	**Day 122:** How to Suck: #1: The Long, Skinny Cock **(158)**	**Day 129:** How to Suck #2: The Short Fat Cock **(166)**
Day 102: The New Side-by-Side Position #1: The Tight Embrace **(134)**	**Day 109:** The PC Factor **(143)**	**Day 116:** The New Missionary Position #2: Crossed Ankles **(151)**	**Day 123:** The Bend-Over Standing Position **(159)**	**Day 130:** The Clitoral Touch **(167)**
Day 103: Playing the Dom **(135)**	**Day 110:** Playing the Submissive **(144)**	**Day 117:** Body Painting **(152)**	**Day 124:** Porn Stars **(160)**	**Day 131:** Breast Intercourse **(168)**
Day 104: Chinese Sex #3: The Swinging Monkey **(138)**	**Day 111:** French Lesson #1: Pompoir (or the Butterfly Quiver) **(145)**	**Day 118:** French Lesson #2: The Parisian Gigolo's Kiss **(153)**	**Day 125:** Advanced Arab Sex #1: Legs in the Air **(161)**	**Day 132:** Advanced Arab Sex #2: Manner of the Bull **(170)**
Day 105: The Ultimate Chakra **(139)**	**Day 112:** New Intimate #1: The Slow Spoon **(146)**	**Day 119:** Expanding Orgasm, Lesson #1 **(154)**	**Day 126:** The Letting-Go Exercise **(162)**	**Day 133:** Slow Sex: Extended Foreplay **(171)**

WEEK 20 A Little More His	WEEK 21 A Sexy Breeze from the East	WEEK 22 Firmer Play	WEEK 23 Easy Moves	WEEK 24 Feel Your Sexual Energy
Day 134: Sexy Yoga, Pose #1 **(172)**	Day 141: Sexy Yoga, Pose #2 **(180)**	Day 148: Sexy Weight Moves #1 **(188)**	Day 155: Sexy Weight Moves #2 **(196)**	Day 162: The Heart Touch **(204)**
Day 135: Small Vibes Quickie **(173)**	Day 142: The Phone Sex Quickie **(181)**	Day 149: The New Kitchen Counter Quickie **(189)**	Day 156: The "Favorite-Friend" Quickie **(197)**	Day 163: The Voyeur Quickie **(205)**
Day 136: How to Suck #3: The BIG Dick **(174)**	Day 143: How to Suck: #4: The Standard Measure **(182)**	Day 150: How to Suck: #5: The Semi-Erect Cock **(191)**	Day 157: The CJ with Hands **(193)**	Day 164: Perineum Orgasm **(206)**
Day 137: The New Missionary Position #3: Open Leg **(175)**	Day 144: No-Fall Release-Him-Now Orgasm **(182)**	Day 151: The Show Masturbation **(192)**	Day 158: The Pressure Orgasm **(200)**	Day 165: Her Multiple Os #2: Sequential **(207)**
Day 138: The Happy Hooker **(176)**	Day 145: The Costume Box **(184)**	Day 152: The Naughty (Male) Nurse **(193)**	Day 159: His Striptease **(200)**	Day 166: Edge Play **(208)**
Day 139: A The Desire Curve **(177)**	Day 146: Indian Sex #1: The Kama Sutra Kiss **(185)**	Day 153: Indian Sex #2: Scratches and Bites **(194)**	Day 160: Indian Sex #3: The Wide-Leg Position **(202)**	Day 167: Japanese Sex #1: Silk and Sake **(209)**
Day 140: Finding God through a Woman's Vagina **(178)**	Day 147: The Red Heels Kiss **(186)**	Day 154: Hearts Breathing **(195)**	Day 161: The Spiritual BJ **(203)**	Day 168: Kundalini #3: Energies Rising Together **(210)**

WEEK 25 Showing Off Your Erotic Skills	WEEK 26 Eclectic Treats	WEEK 27 Sex Writers	WEEK 28 Irresistible Moves	WEEK 29 Coming Together
Day 169: Sharing Grapes (212)	Day 176: Lick an Armpit (220)	Day 183: Sex Journal (228)	Day 190: Simply Irresistible (236)	Day 197: The Snooze Alarm Cuddle (244)
Day 170: "Up-Against-the-Wall" Quickie (213)	Day 177: The Blindfolded Quickie (221)	Day 184: Her Quickie Kit (229)	Day 191: How to Seize The Moment (238)	Day 198: The Call Girl Special (245)
Day 171: "69" with Alternating Tongues (214)	Day 178: The White House BJ Trick (222)	Day 185: Tongue Writing on Her (230)	Day 192: The Historical BJ #4: Josephine's Napoleonic Treat (239)	Day 199: The Figure Eight Lick, Hers (246)
Day 172: The "Go-for-Long" O Tricks (215)	Day 179: His Second Coming (222)	Day 186: The Science of Orgasm (231)	Day 193: Her Multiple Os #3: Serial (240)	Day 200: The New Rear Entry Chest Flat (247)
Day 173: Female Ejaculation (216)	Day 180: Tie and Tease (225)	Day 187: Honey Dust (232)	Day 194: Fingering the Anus (241)	Day 201: Anal Toys, His and Hers (248)
Day 174: Japanese Sex #2: Shunga Sexuality (217)	Day 181: Modifying Your Signature Sex Move (226)	Day 188: Advanced Chinese Sex #1: The Tiger in the Forest Position (233)	Day 195: Advanced Chinese Sex #2: Cicadas Mating (242)	Day 202: Advanced Chinese Sex #3: The Dragon in Flight (249)
Day 175: Expanded Orgasm, Lesson #2 (218)	Day 182: Slow Sex: Start/Stop Thrusting (227)	Day 189: Extragenital Orgasm: The Soul Triggers (234)	Day 196: Face-to-Face Position #2: The Closer Missionary (243)	Day 203: Simultaneous Orgasm, Lesson #1 (250)

WEEK 30 A Little French	WEEK 31 Different Strokes	WEEK 32 Advanced Strokes	WEEK 33 Taking It to the Top	WEEK 34 Surprises for Him
Day 204: The Palm Kiss **(252)**	**Day 211:** Hand/Arm Strokes #1: Feathers **(260)**	**Day 218:** Hand/Arm Strokes #2: Circling Fingers **(268)**	**Day 225:** Hand/Arm Strokes #3: Deep Pressing Fingers **(276)**	**Day 232:** Rub His Chest **(284)**
Day 205: The Gigolo's Delight Quickie **(253)**	**Day 212:** Head of the Penis Quickie Trick **(261)**	**Day 219:** Bathroom Quickie #1: The Nozzle **(269)**	**Day 226:** Bathroom Quickie #2: "Put the Lid Down" **(277)**	**Day 233:** Quickie Dressing **(284)**
Day 206: The French Tickler, Hers **(254)**	**Day 213:** Strumming the Frenulum **(262)**	**Day 220:** The Corona Lick #2 **(270)**	**Day 227:** The Urban BJ #1: Up on the Roof **(278)**	**Day 234:** The Urban CJ #1: Up on the Roof **(285)**
Day 207: The New Sitting Position: Backward Lean **(255)**	**Day 214:** Her Multiple Os #4: Blended **(263)**	**Day 221:** Encouraging Multiple Os **(270)**	**Day 228:** The Surprise Orgasm **(278)**	**Day 235:** Fire Up Your Orgasm **(286)**
Day 208: Anal Intercourse: The Basics **(255)**	**Day 215:** Get Your Laugh On **(264)**	**Day 222:** Anal Intercourse Positions **(271)**	**Day 229:** Create a Secret Life **(281)**	**Day 236:** Meet the Strap-On **(287)**
Day 209: Puritan Sex #2: The White Nightgown **(257)**	**Day 216:** Advanced Indian Sex #1: The Kneeling Man **(265)**	**Day 223:** Advanced Indian Sex #2: The Contrary Position **(273)**	**Day 230:** Advanced Indian Sex #3: Splitting the Bamboo **(282)**	**Day 237:** The Laziest Tantra Position **(288)**
Day 210: Simultaneous Orgasm, Lesson #2 **(258)**	**Day 217:** Simultaneous Orgasm, Lesson #3 **(266)**	**Day 224:** Whole-Body Orgasm **(274)**	**Day 231:** How to Give Her a Whole-Body Orgasm **(283)**	**Day 238:** How to Give Him a Whole-Body Orgasm **(289)**

WEEK 35 Lick Your Yin (or Yang)	WEEK 36 Sexy Whispers	WEEK 37 Sex Management	WEEK 38 Sexy Hearts and Minds	WEEK 39 Building Desire
Day 239: Lick an Instep **(290)**	Day 246: Whisper the Sexy Compliment **(298)**	Day 253: Make the Sexy Suggestion **(306)**	Day 260: Scalp Massage **(314)**	Day 267: The Neck Blow **(322)**
Day 240: The Red Heels Quickie **(291)**	Day 247: The Edge Quickie **(300)**	Day 254: The Time Management Quickie #1: Five Minutes **(307)**	Day 261: The Time-Management Quickie #2: Seven Minutes Five Steps **(315)**	Day 268: The Time-Management Quickie #3: Ten Minutes Five Steps **(323)**
Day 241: The Tut-Tut Suck, Hers **(292)**	Day 248: His Heart in Her Mouth **(301)**	Day 255: The Suburban BJ #1: The Golf Cart **(308)**	Day 262: The Suburban CJ #1: The Sun Roof **(316)**	Day 269: The Bend-Over BJ **(324)**
Day 242: Alternating Orgasms **(294)**	Day 249: The Sensuous Orgasm **(302)**	Day 256: The AFE Zone Orgasms **(310)**	Day 263: Orgasmic Providing **(317)**	Day 270: Visualizing Arousal **(324)**
Day 243: Strap-On Thrusting Techniques **(295)**	Day 250: Role Playing: She's the Boss **(302)**	Day 257: Role Playing: He's The Boss **(311)**	Day 264: Fantasy Exploration **(318)**	Day 271: Thinking Off **(325)**
Day 244: Advanced Japanese Sex #1: The Deep Waters Rear-Entry Position **(296)**	Day 251: Advanced Japanese Sex #2: Lip Service **(303)**	Day 258: Advanced Japanese Sex #3: The Supreme Love Gift **(312)**	Day 265: Lady Libido and the Fire Below **(320)**	Day 272: The Art of Sex **(327)**
Day 245: Discovering Your Yin and Yang Energies **(297)**	Day 252: Cultivating Eclectic Entry #1: The Big Girl's Toy **(305)**	Day 259: Face-to-Face Position #3: Full Flat Female Superior **(313)**	Day 266: Cultivating Eclectic Entry #2: The Big We **(321)**	Day 273: Building the Long Desire: Attraction Plus Obstacles **(328)**

WEEK 40 She Goes Faster	WEEK 41 Deeper Sexual Waters	WEEK 42 Showing Off Her Skills	WEEK 43 From the Naughty to the Sublime	WEEK 44 High Flying
Day 274: The Nipple Rub (330)	**Day 281:** The Lip Pulse Kiss (338)	**Day 288:** The Pelvic Thrust Hug (346)	**Day 295:** Wake up Your Vagina (354)	**Day 302:** The Breast Stroke (362)
Day 275: The Bend-Over Cross Quickie (331)	**Day 282:** The Hands-On Quickie (339)	**Day 289:** The Cowgirl Vibrating Quickie (347)	**Day 296:** No-Panties-Day Quickie (355)	**Day 303:** Movie Quickies #1: *Body Heat* (363)
Day 276: The Cunnilingus Quickie (332)	**Day 283:** The Folded Deck Chair, Hers (340)	**Day 290:** The No-Touch (His Penis) BJ (348)	**Day 297:** The "Make Him Come" BJ (356)	**Day 304:** The Urban BJ #2: The Fire Escape (364)
Day 277: The Sleep Orgasm (332)	**Day 284:** Her Intercourse Orgasm (341)	**Day 291:** It "Sex" If You Don't Orgasm (350)	**Day 298:** Four Easy Steps to Multiple Os (358)	**Day 305:** His G-Spot Orgasm (364)
Day 278: Fantasy Scripts (334)	**Day 285:** The SM Fantasy (342)	**Day 292:** The "Overtaken" Fantasy (351)	**Day 299:** Taking It Out #1: Cuddle Parties (359)	**Day 306:** Taking It Out #2: Sex Club/Sex Party Rules (366)
Day 279: Handling His Desire Curve (336)	**Day 286:** Handling Her Desire Curve (345)	**Day 293:** Dance Lessons #1: Pole Dancing (352)	**Day 300:** Dance Lessons #2: Belly Dancing (360)	**Day 307:** Dance Lessons #3: Dirty Dancing (368)
Day 280: Sex Rituals (337)	**Day 287:** The Long Embrace #1: Karezza (345)	**Day 294:** The Long Embrace #2: Kabazzah (352)	**Day 301:** The Tantra Yab-Yum Position (361)	**Day 308:** The Passion Flower Position (369)

WEEK 45 Passionate Licks	WEEK 46 Higher and Bigger	WEEK 47 Starting with a Kiss Again	WEEK 48 Shoot the Moon	WEEK 49 Flowers and Sex
Day 309: Lick Your Lover's Lips **(370)**	**Day 316:** The Temple Massage **(378)**	**Day 323:** The Eyelid Kiss **(386)**	**Day 330:** The Naked Surprise **(394)**	**Day 337:** Stroke Her with a Flower **(402)**
Day 310: Movie Quickies #2: *The English Patient* **(371)**	**Day 317:** Movie Quickies #3: *Bull Durham* **(379)**	**Day 324:** Movie Quickies #4: *Unfaithful* **(387)**	**Day 331:** Rough Touch Quickie **(395)**	**Day 338:** The Remote-Control Quickie **(403)**
Day 311: The Urban CJ #2: The Fire Escape **(372)**	**Day 318:** The Suburban BJ #2: The Tree House **(379)**	**Day 325:** Oral Sex Positions **(388)**	**Day 332:** The Historical BJ #5: Elizabeth I's Sir Walter Raleigh Special **(395)**	**Day 339:** The Faux Deep Throat **(404)**
Day 312: The Bigger O Trick #1: In Your Hands **(372)**	**Day 319:** The Bigger O Trick #2: Eyes Open/Eyes Closed **(380)**	**Day 326:** The Magic of Ten **(389)**	**Day 333:** The Rule-of-Thumb Orgasm **(398)**	**Day 340:** The Multi-Position Orgasm **(405)**
Day 313: Bringing It In: Your Private Party Rules **(374)**	**Day 320:** Sexual Truth or Dare **(381)**	**Day 327:** The Cum Shot #1: Ejaculating on Breasts **(390)**	**Day 334:** The Cum Shot #2: Giving Her Pearls **(399)**	**Day 341:** Just DO IT **(407)**
Day 314: Dance Lessons #4: Tango **(375)**	**Day 321:** A Tutorial in Classic Porn **(382)**	**Day 328:** Fusion Tantra Position #1: The Moving Sit **(391)**	**Day 335:** The Gentle Chinese Sex Position: The Wedding Night **(400)**	**Day 342:** Sex Online **(408)**
Day 315: Spiritual Sex and Religion **(376)**	**Day 322:** The New Commandments **(384)**	**Day 329:** Sexual/Spiritual Gender Roles **(392)**	**Day 336:** How Much Do You Love Her Pussy/His Cock **(401)**	**Day 343:** The Sexual Puja **(409)**

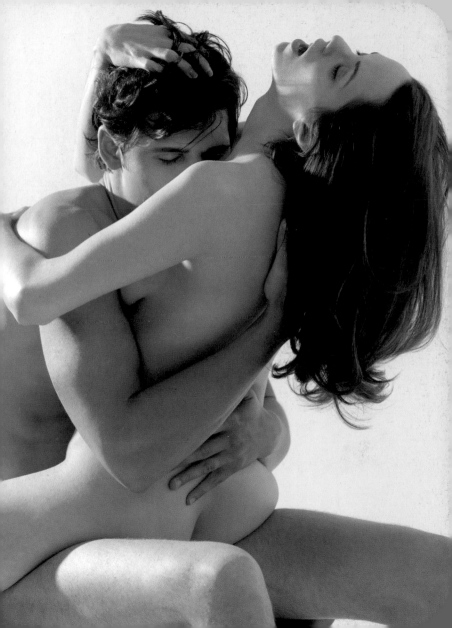

How to Use *Daily Sex Bible*

Has your sex life become a bit too predictable? This book will make it new again, with a different sex tip or technique for every day of the week, each week of the year. You'll get 365 new sex ideas!

I have organized them into theme days:

Flirtation and Foreplay Mondays

Monday is the back-to-work-and-school day—perhaps the least sexy day of the week. Many couples have had sex more than once over the weekend, so they don't feel the strong urge to be sexual on Monday. Sex is not all or nothing. If you put a little sex into the week's real first day, you give the rest of the week added erotic charge. The flirting and foreplay activities—some of which you can do right under the kids' noses—prime you for a quickie the next day, when your sex drive is on the upswing again.

Quickie Tuesdays

Barely into the week, you are caught in the "no time, no energy" trap. It is possible to have quick sex that satisfies both of you (most of the time) and sustains your erotic connection. Sex can be energizing.

Oral Wednesdays

Celebrate Hump Day in a new way. Never mind the happy hour drink specials at the local pub. Take your oral pleasures in one another. You can always pour a little champagne into one another's belly buttons.

Big O Thursdays

The work/school week is almost over. You can stay up a little later on Thursday nights. Go for the bigger, longer, or multiple orgasms.

 Get-Your-Freak-on Fridays

You made it through another week! Dissipate that tension. Go a little wild. The tips and techniques cover everything a vanilla couple wants to know about the other side of sex.

 Sex Ed Saturdays

Part of Saturday is set aside for chores in most families. After you've run through the to-do list, schedule time for adult education and learn about ancient sex, the science of sex, and how to play together at cybersex.

 Spiritual Sundays

Whether you are a churchgoer or not, tap into the spiritual component of your sex life today. Worship one another's bodies and be grateful for the sex life you share.

I hope you will try everything in *Daily Sex Bible*—but do feel free to skip around if a suggestion just doesn't work for you. There's not room in these pages for detailed explanations of sex positions and practices or the science behind sexual behavior. For that, please go to my other bibles: *The Sex Bible*, *The Sex Bible for Women*, and *The Orgasm Bible*.

And I am happy to answer your questions, too. Write to me on my blog at www.sexyprime.typepad.com.

Wishing you at least a little sex in every day,

Susan Crain Bakos

DAY 1: FLIRTATION AND FOREPLAY MONDAY

The "Have A Good Day" Ass Slap

You don't have to look her in the eye while exchanging scheduling information. Pay attention to her ass this morning. A little erotic spanking is part of many couples' sexual repertoire—including yours? Tease her with the hint/promise of more to come later in the week.

As you're both rushing around getting dressed for work, openly admire her beautiful bottom. Reach out and briefly caress it in passing. If you have the opportunity a few minutes later, bend over and plant a quick kiss on one cheek.

When she bends over—and if she doesn't, ask her to bend forward from the waist—cup your hand and lightly slap the other cheek. A cupped hand makes a satisfying sound, one that will stir the erotic senses.

Later when you go your separate morning ways, put your hand over the place you slapped and whisper, "Have a good day, Baby."

....

 DAY 2: QUICKIE TUESDAY

Sex Your Brain

How many times have you read and heard that "sex begins in the brain"? Truly, it does. The brain processes auditory, visual, touch, taste, and scent messages—messages that also trigger sex memories—and mixes up the cocktail of hormones that dilate your pupils, increase your heartbeat and breathing rates, lubricate her vagina, and stiffen his penis. Couples who have been together more than a few years discover that the cocktail doesn't have the same immediate intense impact. But the good news is you can sex your brain by creating rushes of adrenaline and by other means. You have to work that cocktail—especially for a quickie.

Here are some ways of tricking the brain into thinking sex:

Exercise. Can you fit in a lunchtime walk or post-work stop at the gym?

Get scared. Some people are danger junkies because they are addicted to the adrenaline rush. It feels like sex. No time for a rock climb before that quickie? Watch the really scary parts of a scary movie together.

Learn something new. Whether it's the challenge of learning a new job or an online class about writing your memoir, learning excites the brain. Use that excitement as your shuttle bus to sexual desire.

Play "truth or dare." Challenge one another to expose a new layer. Take an unprecedented chance. You don't know everything about each other, you just think you do.

Fall back on the tried-and-true sex tricks. She spends a few minutes alone in the bathroom with her vibrator. He watches some highlights on YouPorn. (Or he strokes himself in the bathroom while she watches the porn.)

Sex that brain—and you'll shake up the cocktail you both need for a good quickie experience.

....

Head Games #1: The New Silken Swirl (incorporating the Butterfly Flick), His

The first third of his penis, including the head, contains the majority of nerve endings. If you can't get the rest of it into your mouth, you can still drive him wild with your BJ technique. You simply need some hot licks for heads, starting with the Silken Swirl, which I learned as a seventeen-year-old reading *The Sensuous Woman* by J. (Thank you, J.) This move could not be simpler—and it's very effective, too.

Continually circle his penis with your tongue while sliding it in and out of your mouth. Pause at the head. Swirl your tongue repeatedly around the head. Now go back to swirling his penis as far as you can take it in, working back to the head, where you will pause again.

Now, before you swirl the shaft again, flick your tongue back and forth lightly across the corona (the ridge between the head and the shaft). Swirl the shaft as far as you can, come back and swirl the head, and flick the corona. Repeat, repeat.

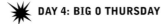

....

💥 **DAY 4: BIG O THURSDAY**

Changing the Orgasm Dynamic

His orgasm is nearly inevitable while hers is often problematic. Why? He comes through friction against the head of the penis, the stimulation he gets during intercourse. But 66 to 75 percent of women need direct clitoral stimulation to reach orgasm—and she probably doesn't get that stimulation from intercourse.

Going back thousands of years to the ancient sexual teachings and continuing today, sex advice aims to change the orgasm dynamic by delaying his ejaculation and speeding her arousal.

How long does it take him to reach orgasm? How long does it take her? Dr. Joel Block, author of *The Art of the Quickie*, says, "On average, four minutes for him, fifteen minutes for her." That eleven-minute differential can be an obstacle to mutually satisfying sex or an opportunity to make sex last longer and feel more intense. Go for the opportunity.

Try this fun exercise today:

1. Make love in your usual way—except don't give her an oral or a manual orgasm before intercourse.

2. Move from foreplay to intercourse when she feels highly aroused.

3. Time his ejaculation.

4. He continues to stimulate her orally, manually, or by stroking her clitoris with the head of his penis.

5. Time her orgasm.

Many of the techniques you'll learn on Big O Thursdays will help delay his ejaculation or increase and intensify her arousal.

. . . .

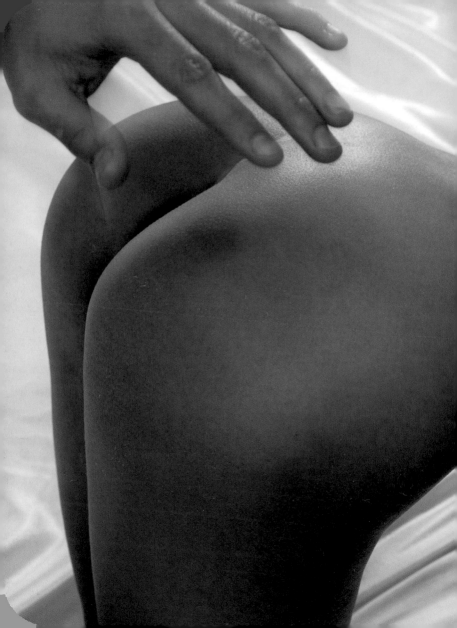

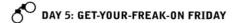 **DAY 5: GET-YOUR-FREAK-ON FRIDAY**

Erotic Spanking

Erotic spanking is a popular activity, particularly among alpha women who welcome the chance to hand over control (temporarily). Done properly, it is delicious foreplay.

How to Spank a Bottom (His or Hers)

From a spanking man: "There aren't many ways to do this. You can start by spanking through fabric, preferably thin panties, to warm up, or you can go straight to the bare flesh. You can cup the hand or not. The flatter your hand, the more intense the sensations. Slap the buttocks, not the middle. Stay away from the smile; go to the cheeks. It's about the anticipation of the blow and the sound when it hits, not usually about corporal punishment. Spank slowly in an irregular, not rhythmic, pattern, so she won't know exactly what is coming next. My secret is to pay attention and continually figure out what my partner likes and give that to her."

And what about the spanking woman? If she can say, "Daddy, I've been a naughty girl"—can't he say, "Mommy, I've been a naughty boy"? Some men enjoy spanking, too. Follow the same directions. A bottom is bottom.

. . . .

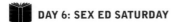 **DAY 6: SEX ED SATURDAY**

Creating Your Signature Sex Move

Most couples have a fallback sex position—the one that *works*, because it's the most all-around satisfying and intimate position for them. Many people also have a signature sex move, the one that seemed to work on every woman/man—or at least we thought it did.

The signature sex move is a good thing (as long as you don't become too dependent on it). Personalizing it to your partner makes it even better. Pay attention to his/her arousal process. What triggers arousal? Heightens it? Encourages orgasm? Or delays it for him? Take that little sex trick, hone it, and make it your signature sex move.

Examples (to get you started):

- The Silken Swirl/Butterfly Flick combination she learned on Wednesday.

- Tip-of-the-Tongue Kissing, using the tip of your tongue to outline one another's lips and tongue—and to dart quickly in and out of mouths.

- The Velvet "No"—a cunnilingus move. He puts his lips around her clitoris, sucks very gently, and with equal subtlety shakes his head from side to side as if he were saying "No."

- Stop/Start Intercourse Moves, designed to delay ejaculation while sustaining arousal. During intercourse, for example, he can vary the speed and depth of thrusting and on a pullout stroke, pause with barely the head of his penis inside her, look into her eyes, and massage her clitoris with his thumb.

....

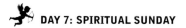 **DAY 7: SPIRITUAL SUNDAY**

The 15-Minute Connection Exercise

Used in acting classes and corporate retreats, this simple exercise helps people overcome the obstacles in their personal relating path without forcing them to endure the jargon of therapeutic expertise. If every time some expert said to "communicate" *and* told you how to do this, I wouldn't hate the word *communicate* so much.

1. Set aside fifteen minutes—all electronics turned off.

2. Stand facing one another. You can clasp hands or not, whatever feels comfortable.

3. Look into one another's eyes and maintain that eye contact for the whole exercise.

4. Consciously regulate your breathing, beginning with deep breaths, until you are breathing in sync.

5. Eye gaze and breathe.

6. You don't have to talk, but you can say whatever you want. For most couples (or exercise participants) the feeling of connection sparks in the first few minutes, and then they are able to speak and listen with their hearts.

....

DAY 8: FLIRTATION AND FOREPLAY MONDAY

Bedtime Story

Ask her to tell you a fantasy as you are holding her in your arms in bed. She probably doesn't want to act out the fantasy as described. You have to pay close attention to her—to who she is, and not just what she's saying. Promise her an erotic fairy tale based on the theme of her fantasy by Friday. You can tell it or read it to her, but do have some scenic elements, such as candles or masks, rose petals or silk ties.

An example:

She fantasizes being raped. The fairy-tale version of that: she is swept off her feet and onto a rose petal–strewn bed by a powerful romantic stranger who satisfies her every desire. Add the specifics. If she has beautiful legs or breasts or a long swanlike neck—whatever she has—focus erotic attention on that.

Having a man pay attention to what a woman says is flattering and very sexy.

....

The Sit-Down-and-Do-It Quickie, His

Sometimes his need is greater than hers (and other times hers is greater than his). Don't play the role of a blowup doll. Take charge of his pleasure. Doing it this way should give you a fair share of your own, too.

Have him sit in a sturdy chair, preferably one without arms or a wide padded chair with room for her legs on the sides. Take off your skirt and panties and make sure he has a good view.

Hand him a small vibe to use on your clitoris.

Unzip his pants, take out his penis, and pay a little attention to it as he strokes your clitoris.

Sit down on his penis. You can fold your legs to the sides of him, or, if the chair permits, keep your feet on the floor. Either way, you have leverage, either by rocking up and down on thigh power or by using your feet.

While you control the thrusting, he works the vibe.

Maintain intense eye contact with him. Your hands are free to caress his face or tweak his nipples. How you handle your man sets the tone for this as a tender or tough and hot experience.

....

The Whiskey Dick Cunnilingus Technique, Hers

Sometimes a man is too tired for intercourse. Or he's had too much to eat or drink to perform well. Dave B. has been in restaurant management in Manhattan for twenty years, which means long hours, late nights, free drinks, and sometimes "a whiskey dick." After age thirty, he says, every man needs to perfect his oral game because eventually, for one reason or another, his penis will let him down.

From Dave B.:

1. Lick her slow and easy until she starts getting wet and silky.

2. Now do the A move: Go down one side of the clitoris and then down the other, gently sucking on each side as gently as you can. You want the tip of the clit to pop out of the hood, so keep making the A until it does.

3. Then use the swirl, circling her clit with the tip of your tongue.

4. Now try the Z move: Lick across the top, slant down the shaft, and lick across the bottom.

5. When she is crazy for it, thrust the tip of your tongue fast—not hard—on the tip of her clit (or the sides, if the tip is too sensitive).

6. Practice, practice, practice.

....

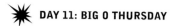 **DAY 11: BIG O THURSDAY**

The Venus Butterfly

Bob and Leah Schwartz, authors of *The One-Hour Orgasm: How to Learn the Amazing "Venus Butterfly,"* gave this technique its name—reputedly lifted from an episode of an 80s TV show, *L.A. Law*—but the technique itself actually dates back to the 1960s, when Lafayette Morehouse created a commune in California dedicated to sexuality. Most manual techniques for giving a woman an orgasm that are taught in sex workshops are based on the Morehouse method.

1. His hands are clean, nails trimmed—and fingers lubed.

2. She lies down; he sits beside her.

3. Placing one hand under hips, he curves the other hand at the top of her mons, so his middle finger can easily reach down to stroke her clitoris.

4. With the thumb or fingers of his lower hand, he gently parts her labia.

5. With the middle finger of his top hand, he strokes up and down around the clitoral area. (Bob Schwartz says, "Imagine your finger as a delicate butterfly wing.") Keep reapplying lube as necessary.

....

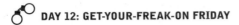 **DAY 12: GET-YOUR-FREAK-ON FRIDAY**

The Lady in Pearls

Are you ready to act out a fantasy based on her bedtime story from Monday night? If not, I have one to inspire you.

The gentleman is waiting in the room when the lady arrives. He smiles and nods approvingly at her. As she slips off her coat, he sees that she is wearing nothing but black stockings, red heels, and strands of pearls—and his smile widens. He has always liked a lady in pearls.

He undresses and sits on the edge of the bed. She goes to her knees and takes his cock firmly in one hand. It swells to her touch. As she bends her head to him, one long strand of pearls slide down over his cock. She takes the pearls between two fingers of the hand holding his cock and gently rubs them up down, following them with her tongue. He sees faint traces of her red lipstick on his shaft in the wake of her skillful mouth—and this excites him more. She plays his cock until he feels ready to burst. His hands on her head are insistent, guiding her to take him all the way into her mouth. Gasping, he pulls her hair.

She wraps the pearls around his balls and tugs upward. After he shoots his cum down her throat, he realizes that his balls are throbbing. He pulls her hair again. She loosens the strand of pearls around his balls . . .

But in a short while, she will show him what else she can do with those pearls.

....

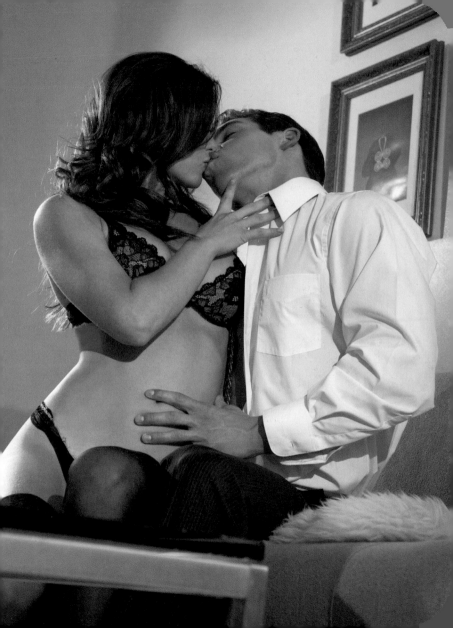

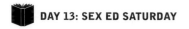

Arab Sex #1:
The Cavalier on Horseback

No, Arab sex is not doing it in the dark through a hole in her burka. *The Perfumed Garden*, the bible of that branch of Eastern sex, was written in the sixteenth century, when Arab civilization led the world in culture and intellectual achievement. The author was a scholar, Sheik Umar ibn Muhammad al-Nafzawi. His ruler, the Grand Vizier to the Bay of Tunis, commissioned him to write a manual on the arts of love. That great erotic explorer Sir Richard Burton translated the book into English in the nineteenth century.

This simple twist on the man-on-top position changes the coital dynamics, and the sensations are fantastic. She feels deliciously submissive and "taken" by her powerful riding man. Her hands are free to stimulate her clitoris. He can last longer in this variation than in most versions of the missionary.

1. She lies on her back with her legs crossed above the ankles, tucked loosely under her calves. Her folded legs elevate her vulva, making connection with her G-spot and clitoral stimulation more likely—and none of his weight is on her.

2. He straddles her, with his legs on either side of her, weight on his knees.

3. He rides her "like a cavalier on horseback," sometimes leaning slightly forward, sometimes back.

············

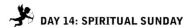 **DAY 14: SPIRITUAL SUNDAY**

Soul Kissing

In the beginning of a relationship, couples kiss a lot. As time goes on, they kiss less and less. But kissing is an intrinsic part of good sex. We taste, touch, and smell our lovers in a deep sensual kiss.

To put the soul back into kissing, each person should:

- Keep your eyes open at least part of the time.

- Lead with the tip of your tongue. "Deep" kissing does not mean ramming your tongue down her (or his) throat.

- Play with your lover's lips with the tip of your tongue and then circle his tongue with the tip of yours—again and again.

- Thrust the tip of your tongue in and out of her mouth as you caress her face and play with her hair.

- Tease one another with tongue play as you run your hands up and down each other's bodies.

- Circle the tip of his tongue as if it were the head of his penis.

- Pull back once or twice to gently lock lips and look into one another's eyes—and pick up the tempo again.

....

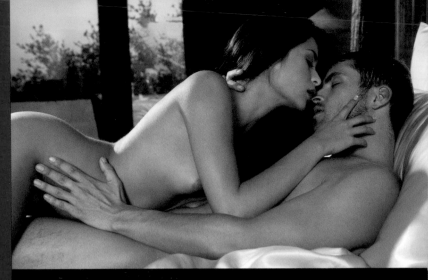

👁 DAY 15: FLIRTATION AND FOREPLAY MONDAY

The Nuzzle Rub

You don't have to do this one behind the children's backs. Nuzzling is sexy between grown-ups—but it looks innocent to the little ones.

1. Put your hands on his (or her) shoulders and use your finger pads to massage some of the tension away.

2. As you're doing this, nuzzle the back of his head. If she (or he) has long hair, briefly bury your face in it.

3. Keep massaging and nuzzling your lover's neck.

4. Wrap up your mini massage with a neck kiss.

....

The Gift-Wrapped Quickie, Hers

If you haven't played with bondage tape, you've been missing out on the fun. I love the pink stuff. You can wrap it around your breasts and ass in the most flattering ways. (The tape lifts as well as binds!) A roll of pink tape can amp up any sex act. The secret: Treat it like gift wrap, not the all-purpose duct tape that you use around the house.

He needs to do a little advance planning. If she doesn't own a waterproof vibe, order one. And, of course, don't forget the tape.

1. Toward the end of her bath or shower, hand her a waterproof vibe and tell her to stop just before she comes.

2. As she's toweling off, surprise her with a roll of pink bondage tape.

3. Start wrapping her up in the bathroom. Lead her to the bedroom to finish. Be creative—but make sure you wrap her wrists and leave her legs open for pleasure.

4. As she is resting comfortably on her back, kneel in front of her open legs. Use the vibe on her clitoris until she is writhing and begging to come. (Under two minutes. Really.)

5. You can either wrap her legs around your neck or position her feet against your chest—or put one leg around your neck and leave the other one, knee bent, foot on the bed. Each of these variations helps her reach orgasm, especially when you have her so turned on—you're just driving it home.

....

The Oral/G-Spot Double Play, Hers

This has nothing to do with baseball. But the name does appeal to a sports-loving man, doesn't it?

As you are licking and sucking her clitoris and the surrounding area, add this G-spot stroke:

1. Insert a finger or two into her vagina and massage her G-spot (see page 66 for how to find it).

2. Try tapping it repeatedly with your fingertip.

3. Rub the spot if she doesn't respond to the tapping. Alternate broad strokes with circular rubbing.

4. Flick your tongue rapidly around her clitoris as you're massaging her G-spot. Don't be surprised if she "ejaculates" during this orgasm.

....

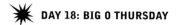 **DAY 18: BIG O THURSDAY**

The Long Tease

Men who have watched a lot of porn often think that sex is hard-driving from start to finish. (Sometimes it is, but not usually.) As soon as she's aroused, they move out of the foreplay stage and into driver mode. Women love to be teased sexually. You can bring a woman to a strong orgasm or a series of multiples by teasing.

Play with her, both orally and manually. When she is very aroused, pull back. Dial down the stimulation. Bring her up, let her back down—over and over again, until she's begging for release. Don't let her come until she does beg.

For example, stop cunnilingus before orgasm. Hold her and stroke her breasts or thighs until her arousal subsides. Back to the cunnilingus. Stop again.

Stroke her, this time moving from nongenital caresses to her labia and finally playing with her clitoris. Stop again.

Repeat oral and manual teasing as desired.

The slow build creates enormous erotic tension, leading to an explosive release.

....

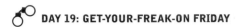

The "Do Me" Appointment

It's been a long week. If he (or she) has a private office, call and tell him you're leaving work early and will meet him there. No office? Create one at home.

Be inspired by this woman's story:

"I need you," I said. "I need you inside me now."

"I'm in a meeting, but I can be free in thirty minutes," he said.

When I got there, he was alone in his office. He loosened his tie as he walked toward me.

"Do me," I begged.

My fingers trembled as I unbuttoned his shirt; I needed to inhale his chest and feel the curly hair on my face. He unzipped my skirt. I'd already removed my panties in the cab. (Now you know why I've never been a pantyhose kind of gal.) We are expert at the semi-dressed fuck.

He scooped me up and carried me to the leather sofa. The man is big and powerful, in more than one sense of the word. While kissing me passionately, he caressed my vulva, penetrated my vagina with two fingers, and circled his thumb around my clit. I was ready to be fucked almost immediately—and he didn't keep me waiting.

He did me. I needed it so bad.

....

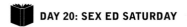

Arab Sex #2:
The Short Penis Position

Don't turn the page! Even if your penis isn't short, you can still enjoy this position and give her a lot of pleasure. It also works if your erection is not as hard as it usually is. And it's a great position for teasing her by inserting only the first third of your penis, pulling it out every other stroke, and rubbing the head against her clitoris. That will drive her crazy. This is the second of eleven classic Arab intercourse positions, from *The Perfumed Garden*:

1. She lies on her back.

2. Lift her legs up and over her shoulders as far as is comfortable for her. (Place a pillow under her buttocks to help her sustain the position.) The closer her legs are to her ears, the more her vulva pushes forward.

3. He kneels between her legs. His short penis feels like it is thrusting more deeply inside her.

The Arabs understood that women need more time in lovemaking to reach orgasm than men do. Their sexual practices included oral and manual foreplay for her. The intercourse positions were designed to maximize her clitoral stimulation and help him delay his ejaculation.

....

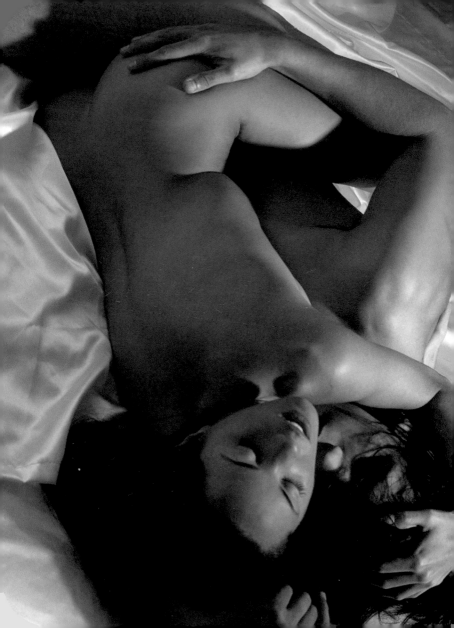

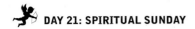 **DAY 21: SPIRITUAL SUNDAY**

Sensual Caressing

Linger as long as possible under the sheets before getting up to make breakfast. Take turns caressing one another. The partner receiving the caresses closes his or her eyes to focus solely on physical sensation.

In a side-by-side position, the giver lies on one side and glides (lightly oiled or creamed) hands in big motions from the neck down over the breasts (chest), belly, thighs, and legs.

Facing one another in a full-body embrace, the giver uses big, gliding strokes down the lover's back, gently cups and caresses each buttock, softly kneads each one in turn, and uses finger pads in a pressing caress up the spine.

In a spoon position, with the receiver's back against the giver's front, the receiver uses the flats of his or hands to caress/rub the chest or breasts and takes the movement down the body, covering the belly and thighs.

. . . .

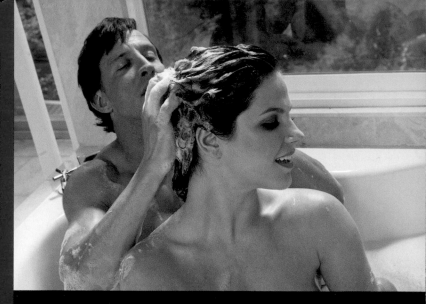

👁 **DAY 22: FLIRTATION AND FOREPLAY MONDAY**

Surprise Back Scrub

The morning rush can be so programmed that one partner puts on the coffee (or changes the baby) while the other showers. They pass one another going in and out of the bathroom on the shift change. Today, design your shift to overlap slightly with your partner's.

Slip into the bathroom while she or he is in the shower. Suds up a cloth, sponge, or loofah and give your lover a leisurely back scrub. End with a few swirling motions around the buttocks.

Hurry back to your domestic post.

. . . .

The Hand-Job Quickie, His

Every now and then, in the course of a committed relationship, someone gives it up for the sake of the other. You may regard this as a credit in the sex bank, meaning the next "quid" in quid pro quo is yours. Or you may realize that a lover's gratitude is its own reward. Using four easy moves, you can make him SO happy.

As he's pressing his erection against you and begging for attention, whisper in his ear, "I'll give you five minutes."

Unzip his pants and take that big boy out. Lube your hands. Clasp them together, fingers laced, snugly around the shaft of his penis.

In #1, move your hands up the shaft in one long twisting motion. Repeat the twisting upward move, picking up speed with the repetitions.

For #2, move your hands to the top of the shaft. Gently squeeze, contract and release, at one-second intervals.

In #3, cradle his balls in one hand and grasp the shaft with the other, moving it upward in a single continuous motion. When you get to the head, rotate your hand slightly in a jar-opening motion.

Finish with #4. Take his shaft firmly in both hands and work it up and down quickly—as you've seen him do it when he masturbates.

You can take his head into your mouth and swallow his cum—or watch him ejaculate.

. . . .

Dirty Talk to the Pussy

Talk to her while you're going down on her. She won't be able to understand anything you say. That's not the point. This is a different kind of communication. The vibrations from your voice and the unpredictability of those tremors will make her come even quicker.

Say all the dirty things you might not feel comfortable saying—or she hearing—in her ear. (Just knowing what you're saying down there will increase your excitement level, too.)

Use your nose to rub on and around her clitoris while you're talking. The nose makes an excellent clitoral stimulator, giving her different sensations than your tongue. (At last, men with big noses can get respect.)

....

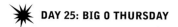 **DAY 25: BIG 0 THURSDAY**

Breath Orgasms: Nan Wise's Suspended Breath and Extended Exhalation

A therapist/coach, neuroscience researcher, and student/teacher of yoga, Tantra, and other disciplines, Nan Wise shares her secrets for making orgasm more intense through breathing techniques.

Suspended Breath

As you build up to orgasm, stall your breath. Take a shallow inhalation—inhale but don't "overfill" your lungs—and hold it, then let it out slowly. Keep doing this for several seconds. It should feel like you are in a place of stalled breathing because you are inhaling and exhaling small amounts of air.

Extended Exhalation

Next, suspend exhalation—or, in other words, hold your breath. When you are almost at orgasm, take a deep breath. As you feel the orgasm begin, exhale in a big, extended breath while imagining sparks flying out of your vagina (or penis). The exhalation should extend and expand your orgasm.

....

The Forbidden Lick

This tip comes from Master J, one of the interesting characters I've met in Maxie's Grill, a Gramercy Park bar in Manhattan. Master J was part of the scene in the days of Plato's Retreat, Hellfire, and other S&M clubs. He knows how to please women, often by giving them something they secretly crave—like analingus.

The anus is rich in nerve endings. Playing there does seem naughty or even taboo—and that ratchets up arousal.

From J: "Men want anal intercourse. Many women don't want that, but they secretly desire another kind of attention to their asshole. They want to be licked. Lick her asshole; rim it with your tongue and then your finger. 'Fuck' it with just the tip of your tongue then the tip of your finger."

Caveat: If her asshole isn't "lickable" clean, she'll be embarrassed—and you likely won't be so happy either after you swallow some unwelcome bacteria. Shower or bathe together first. Suds up her bottom and gently use a washcloth-covered finger around and slightly into her anus. An added safety measure: a piece of plastic wrap between tongue and anus.

....

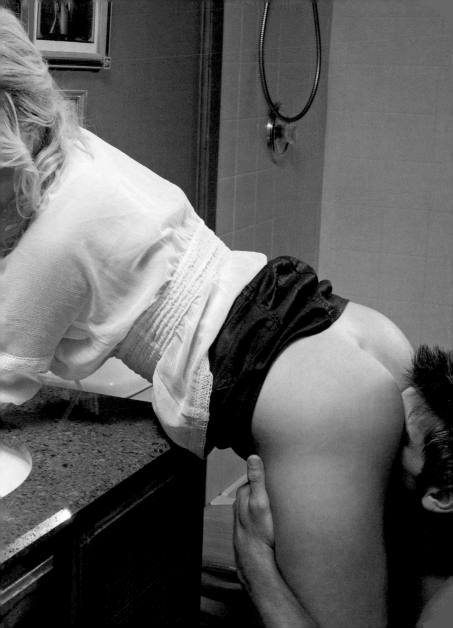

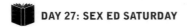 **DAY 27: SEX ED SATURDAY**

Sex Trick:
Keeping a "Fall-Out" Penis Inside

Every couple experiences the same (or similar) little annoying technical problems from time to time. They can be easily tuned up. This Saturday, extend your "fix it" mode to sex.

What causes penis fall-out? Fast thrusting, and positions that need adjusting to accommodate a particular penis.

1. Men, slow down. The jackhammer approach to intercourse is mainly effective in porn as a tool for your arousal.

2. Women, grab his ass, hold it, and control his rhythm by lightly squeezing his buttocks when you want him to thrust.

3. Two positions provide the deepest penetration: rear entry and missionary (or man on top)—if she puts her legs up on his shoulders. Depending on your relative sizes and flexibility, she may rest her ankles or the backs of her calves against his shoulders.

4. The most fall-out probably occurs when she's on top. Try moving in a circular fashion rather than up and down or back and forth; however, some men find that circling uncomfortable.

5. Make sure you do sets of supereasy Kegel exercises three or four times a week to keep your PC (vaginal floor) muscle firm. See page 143.

....

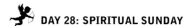 **DAY 28: SPIRITUAL SUNDAY**

A Penis Altar

The phallus was openly venerated in many cultures. We in the modern West erect more subtle shrines to the phallus, such as the Washington Monument.

In ancient Egypt, Japan, and Greece, among other societies, the phallus was a fertility symbol. The Romans wore phallic-shaped jewelry as talismans to ward off the evil eye. In India, the god Shiva is still often represented by a phallic symbol known as the lingam. And every year National Penis Day is celebrated in Japan.

Suggestions for your penis altar:

- Statues of Priapus, fertility god and son of Aphrodite, and other Greek and Roman phallic symbols

- Brass trinkets—key chains and small figures of men with outsize erections—from African and Indian shops

- Drawings, paintings, or sketches of the penis

- Candles, incense, small bud vases for flowers

- If you don't want obvious phallic symbols, display a lingam, which looks like a round piece of sculpture with a flat bottom, like a pillar candle more than a cock. You can find nice ones in marble, brass, and wood. Surround it with the candles, incense, and flowers.

- No matter what anyone says, a man wants his cock worshipped, and women who worship the cock get what they want in the end.

. . . .

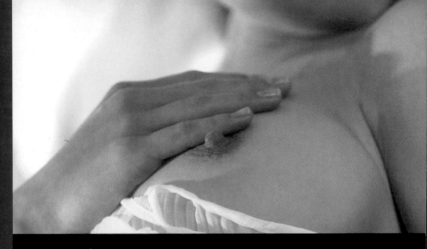

DAY 29: FLIRTATION AND FOREPLAY MONDAY

Seducing the Nipple

She's wearing a silk blouse or cotton T-shirt. The suit jacket hasn't been layered on yet. If her bra is sheer enough, you can see her nipples. But you want to see them stand up before you rush off to work.

Seduce the nipple by "accidentally" brushing her breast with your arm or hand:

• Stand very close to her as you make innocuous conversation.

• Look into her eyes, take a heavy breath, and caress her cheek.

• Let your hand trail down her throat and breast.

• Palm her nipple, press lightly, and blow on her neck.

....

The Hand-Job Quickie, Hers

Sometimes she's gotta have it, and you're too tired or time-challenged. This hand-job quickie, augmented by the vibe of your choice, will satisfy her and make you feel like the noble, generous lover that you are. Bonus: You get to watch.

1. Rub lube into your hands. Using a firm touch, caress her thighs in an upward stroke that blends into her genitals. Part her lips with your fingers and stroke her inner labia.

2. *Surround* her clitoris with your thumb and forefinger, but don't squeeze it! Massage gently.

3. If she likes having her clitoris stroked directly, do that now. Try varying strokes by holding it between thumb and forefinger and lightly rotating.

4. Hold two fingers in the shape of a V and put them around her clitoris. Press down lightly. Pull back. Press down again and back up, creating a rocking motion that may bring her to orgasm.

5. If needed, turn on a vibe designed for external use—and let her hip movements guide you.

....

The Historical BJ #1:
Catherine the Great's Special

According to reputable historians, those rumors about Catherine and horses were not true. Queen of Russia in the 1700s, she and her husband, Peter, expanded the empire, supported the development of the arts, and Westernized the court. Both had many lovers. Catherine reputedly enjoyed performing fellatio on her lovers and was said to be quite skilled at it.

How would a powerful woman with a short attention span perform a blow job? Maybe like this:

1. Put a big floor pillow between his legs and sink gracefully to your knees. (Powerful women like to play at being submissive sometimes.)

2. Take his cock into both hands as you gaze adoringly at *it*, not him. Inhale him from head to balls.

3. Begin with slow, broad licks up the shaft. Keep one hand busy with his balls while working his shaft with the other.

4. With the tip of your tongue, outline the corona, the ridge separating the head from the shaft. Now swirl your tongue around the head. Swirl and lick. Alternate with sucking as much of the shaft as you can comfortably take into your mouth.

5. Pick up your pace as he grows more excited. Take that hand off his balls and put it on your clit. You come, too. Would a queen give without getting?

....

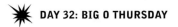 **DAY 32: BIG O THURSDAY**

The A-Frame Effect

This is another cunnilingus tip from Dave B. (who may soon find himself in need of a social secretary to book his dates).

He says, "If her clitoral shaft is too sensitive to touch after an orgasm or two, switch to the A-frame. You're sustaining her arousal so she can come again and again—without making her uncomfortable."

The area just above the clitoral shaft is the tip of the A. Form the sloping sides of the letter A by tracing the tip of your tongue from the top of the A down the surrounding tissue on either side. The line forms right under the shaft.

Trace that A, top to bottom, slowly. Repeat several times. Pick up the pace.

Now trace it, bottom to top, several times, again slowly, followed by faster repetitions.

Mix it up. Trace one leg of the A, then a side, the line, and the other side. Keep mixing it up as you change up the pace.

. . . .

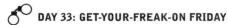

Painting Her O

The late actress Farrah Fawcett was also an artist. In her fifties, with a still-spectacular body, she created some memorable body art by covering herself in paint and making love to big sheets of white paper spread on the floor.

Inspired by Farrah, paint your orgasm.

1. Put a clear plastic tarp down. Place large sheets of white paper on top of that.

2. Using edible body paints (or real paints, if you want a lasting memento), paint her body.

3. As you're painting her, she masturbates, with a vibe or without.

4. When she is close to orgasm, she simulates an intercourse position with the paper, rubbing against it to induce the O.

The results will amaze you.

....

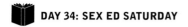 **DAY 34: SEX ED SATURDAY**

Arab Sex #3: The Art of Brinksmanship

The art of brinkmanship is the man's ability to pull himself back from the ejaculatory edge. Some men train themselves to do this repeatedly during intercourse so they can stay highly aroused for longer periods of time without ejaculating. A few men claim they can experience orgasm without ejaculation through complete mastery of brinksmanship.

A more modest goal: Extend intercourse a little longer. Here's how to do it:

1. Practice while masturbating, when you can focus entirely on your own process of arousal.

2. Continue stimulation to the point of near orgasm. Stop.

3. Don't resume stimulation until your arousal level has declined.

4. Repeat as often as possible. Your orgasm should feel stronger—an added benefit.

. . . .

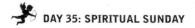

The Legend of the Lingam

The Hindu god Shiva is represented by the lingam, the subtle phallus symbol that (as previously noted) looks more like a pillar candle than a cock.

The lingam has its roots in a formless concept of god, before Shiva and the other gods and goddesses were created from the vortex. Once he was given a form, Shiva declared that he was one with his phallus. The Hindus drew a central belief from that: The phallus is the foundation of life. Shiva, they say, ordered veneration of the lingam.

Some of the megalithic monuments to Shiva still standing in modern India are thousands of years old. They remind us that the lingam (together with the yoni) create life—but it is interesting to note that Shiva and his consorts Shakti, Parvati, and Sati did not procreate. Their expanded definition of the life force should appeal to citizens of the twenty-first century who rarely procreate but often mate.

"The phallus is the source of pleasure," Shiva also said. "Every orgasm is a divine experience."

Worship together at the penis altar (see page 51). Now she falls to her knees and worships his cock in the manner most pleasing to him.

....

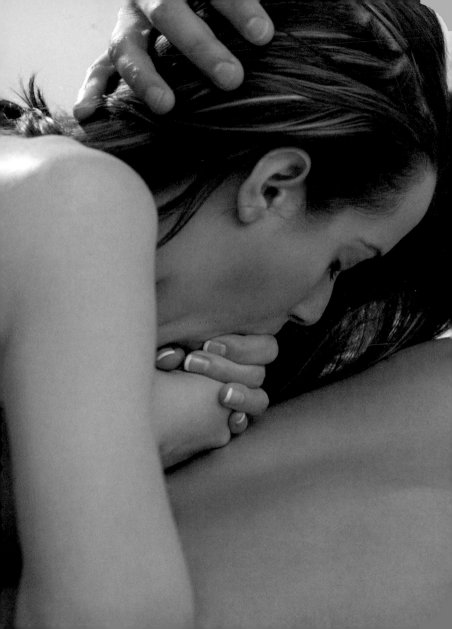

DAY 36: FLIRTATION AND FOREPLAY MONDAY

Thigh-High Kissing

As you're getting dressed, either for work or for a social engagement, pull on a pair of sexy lace-topped thigh-high stockings. Put on your heels and walk around the bedroom in your bra, panties, and thigh-highs. Now that you have his attention...

Perch on the edge of the bed or a chair.

Tell him to "come here."

Ask him, "Will you kneel down and kiss my thighs?"

Open your legs and show him where you want to be kissed by running a finger along each inner thigh.

When he has kissed you well on both thighs, take his face in your hands, kiss his mouth, thank him—and get up and finish dressing.

....

The Morning Quickie

There are so many reasons *not* to have sex in the morning: No time for the foreplay or the cleanup. No privacy. One of you is not a morning person. But it feels so good . . .

Here's one way of doing it:

Before you fall asleep the night before, kiss and caress one another.

Set your alarm for ten minutes earlier than usual. Put the clock on his side of the bed.

If one of you wakes in the night, caress (without waking) the other.

When the alarm goes off, he slides beneath the sheets and gives her an oral wake-up call.

Within minutes, she will pull him up and take him inside.

. . . .

The Clitoral Roots, an Anatomy Lesson

You probably know that the clitoris is the only organ on the human body designed solely for pleasure—but did you know that the little pink shaft and surrounding hood are only part of the clitoris? The clitoris has 8,000 nerve endings and operates within a network of 15,000 nerve endings that service the entire pelvic region. Thus, all orgasms are really clitoral—even if the little pink shaft receives no direct stimulation. Here are the parts of that most amazing female organ:

- The clitoral hood: A small outgrowth (or overgrowth) of skin covering the clitoral glans or shaft. When a woman becomes aroused, the shaft protrudes from the hood, though in some women just barely.

- The clitoral glans or shaft: It is so incredibly sensitive because the vast system of nerves connecting the clitoris to the vagina all end *here*.

- The crura (a.k.a. wings): Crura look like the legs of a wishbone. Located to the right and left of the urethra, they run back to the pubic bone and connect to the clitoris at the point of the inverted, or upside down, V.

- The vestibular or clitoral bulbs: This string of bulb-shaped aggregations of erectile tissue extends down beneath the labia minora, or inner lips. During arousal, they fill with blood, making the vulva swell.

- Front commissure: A very sensitive and often overlooked area above the base of the clitoral shaft, just below where the labia majora, or outer lips, meet.

....

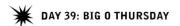 **DAY 39: BIG O THURSDAY**

The New Woman on Top #1:
The Shy Reverse Cowgirl

Her butt is a hard area for a woman to love. Some women even walk backward out of a room if they are naked. Many won't even try the Reverse Cowgirl because they don't want their butt that close to his face. This tip from a regular SexyPrime reader (a woman who "hates" her butt) might just change their minds.

Dress for It

If you have the money and inclination, buy a latex cat suit with a genital opening. What a butt shaper! Or buy a pair of Spanks panties and create an opening.

Or wear an oversized black silk shirt or one of his white shirts, open at the front, and let it settle over your ass as you ride.

Or put on a bustier with garters that wrap around your buttocks and hold up your flesh as they hold up your stockings.

Lean Forward

When you lean forward, you smooth out the pockets and wrinkles in your buttocks. Bonus: better clitoral stimulation.

Move Vigorously

If you thrust fast and furious, he won't be studying the dimples in your ass.

....

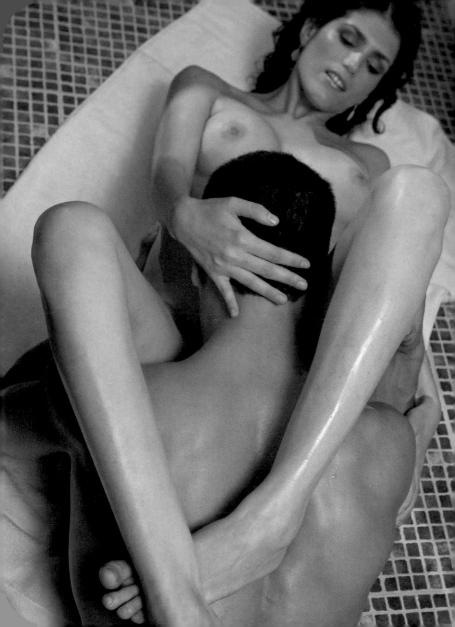

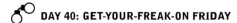 **DAY 40: GET-YOUR-FREAK-ON FRIDAY**

The Roman Romp

The Romans held some of their fabled orgies in the lavish public baths. Food was an essential part of every sex party. Your bathroom may be humble, but you can still hold an orgy for two in there. Light candles. Wrap yourselves in shawls or scarves. Bring in the wine (or better yet, champagne), trays of fruit (don't forget the grapes), cheese, and bread—and that delight unknown to Romans, the waterproof vibe.

Try:

• Perfuming the water

• Eating grapes out of her pussy

• Drizzling honey over his cock

• Using the vibe on her clitoris in the rear-entry position

• Feeding one another with your mouths

• Drinking champagne from one another's belly buttons

• Covering the toilet in a lovely cloth, calling it a throne, and letting the courtesan ride the emperor

• Taping the gladiator's hands over his head to the bathroom wall and letting the noble lady ravish him

• Feasting and copulating 'til dawn

. . . .

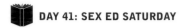 **DAY 41: SEX ED SATURDAY**

Questing for G-Spots, His and Hers

Interestingly, the debate on whether her G-spot exists rages on—while the conventional wisdom acknowledges his. Men, no excuses: Look for it.

How to Find Her G-Spot (and What to Do When You Have)

Thousands of years ago, the authors of the Kama Sutra wrote about the G-spot. Rediscovered in modern times, the G-spot is a small mass of rough tissue about a third of the way up the front vaginal wall. In some women, it swells when stimulated and produces orgasm.

Take your hand, palm up, to the opening of her vagina. Insert two fingers and make the "come hither" gesture. Do you feel a difference in the texture of the skin? Stroke it with your finger, tap on it with a finger pad, or use a special G-spot vibe on it.

How to Find His G-Spot (and What to Do When You Have)

His G-spot is located inside the body behind the perineum. You can reach it in two ways: by pressing the perineum with your thumb or finger, and by inserting a finger into his anus and using the same "come hither" gesture that he used in your vagina.

Stroking the perineum from the inside can drive some men wild—and does nothing for others. Likewise, pressing your thumb into his perineum may induce orgasm/ejaculation—or not.

G-spots—not an exact science. But when they work, they really work.

....

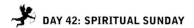 **DAY 42: SPIRITUAL SUNDAY**

A Pussy Altar

Worship of female genitalia goes back thousands of years. Goddess and earth-based religions venerated the vulva. The Divine Woman even appeared in cave paintings, her legs open, exposing her vulva for all to adore.

In modern times, the yoni (vulva) is still worshipped in the Hindu faith. But in the West, self-proclaimed "goddesses" tend to be a narrower group: older white women into Tantra or some other form of Eastern sexual mysticism. That's too bad. Let's expand pussy worship to make it more attractive to all of us. Power to the pussy! Where would the world be without it?

Some suggestions for your pussy altar:

- Orchids!—yes, the flower that inspired Georgia O'Keefe—either sprays in water or plants

- Paintings, drawings, or sketches of the vulva

- Vulva sculptures

- Candles, flowers, incense

- For a more subtle altar, display a yoni, which is round with a flat base and an indentation in the center—much like a candleholder created for the lingam. You can buy them in Indian shops.

. . . .

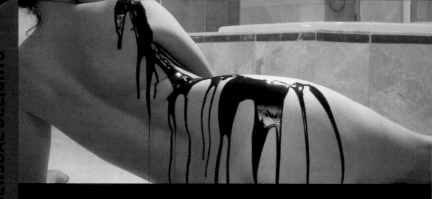

DAY 43: FLIRTATION AND FOREPLAY MONDAY

Tantalizing the Taste Buds

When you excite one of the senses, you make the others more easily aroused, too. A new and thrilling taste can make you want to experience a different kind of touch. Feed one another bites of new foods. Lick off fingers and lips. Try:

- Dark chocolate with chile pepper
- Fried oysters
- Raspberry jam (pure fruit, no added sugar)
- French fries covered in melted blue cheese
- Cashew butter

- Nutella
- Exotic truffles
- Hot bread dripping in honey butter
- Green tea ice cream
- Mango chutney
- Fresh figs

Buy *InterCourses: An Aphrodisiac Cookbook* by Martha Hopkins and Randall Lockridge—and make a new dish together.

....

Redefining "Sex"

"Sex" can be:

- Flirting
- Touching
- Kissing
- Caressing
- Oral genital stimulation, for one or both
- Manual genital stimulation, for one or both
- Intercourse
- Anal play
- Anal intercourse
- Mutual masturbation
- And what else? Can you add to the list?

Although we usually think of a quickie as fast intercourse, it can also be an oral or a manual experience—or mutual masturbation. Think of all the ways you can satisfy each other—or one bring the other to orgasm—in a short space of time. Make a quickie wish list.

. . . .

The Corona Lick #1

The corona is the ridge separating the head of the penis from the shaft. This highly sensitive place is generally a favored licking spot in fellatio. Today, make it the central focus of your BJ—right up to the point where he needs suction to bring him to orgasm.

1. Begin with the routine strokes, running the flat of your tongue up and down the shaft, outlining the corona and head with the tip of your tongue, swirling your tongue around the head.

2. Circle the corona rapidly and repeatedly with the tip of your tongue.

3. Slowly lick it.

4. Alternate the flicking and licking.

5. Take the head and corona into your mouth and suck.

....

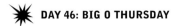 **DAY 46: BIG O THURSDAY**

Her Multiple Os #1:
Compounded Single Orgasms

Physiologically, all women are capable of multiple orgasms because women have no refractory period between one orgasm and another. There are four types of female multiple orgasms: compounded singles (the most common), sequential multiples, serials, and blended multiples. Each orgasm is distinct, separated by sufficient time so that prior arousal and tension have substantially resolved between orgasms.

How to have compounded single orgasms:

1. Stop clitoral stimulation when the first orgasm begins. Move stimulation to the sides of the clitoris (or to the labia if the entire clitoral area is momentarily too sensitive for touch).

2. As the orgasm subsides, stimulate the clitoris (or surrounding area) again, using an alternate method—for example, if the first orgasm resulted from oral stimulation, use your hand. Or switch vibe speeds and positions—even switch vibes.

3. After the second orgasm, go back to the first form of stimulation. Be sensitive to what is working. Keep changing it up.

. . . .

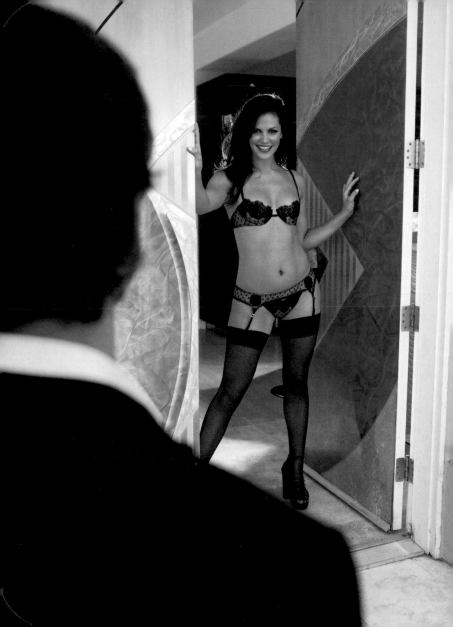

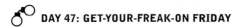 **DAY 47: GET-YOUR-FREAK-ON FRIDAY**

Her Striptease

You don't need a perfect body to strip for your man. Nor must you take it *all* off. Show off your best parts and finish with a presentation of your pussy.

Preparation

- Practice stripping to your favorite music.

- Have a glass of wine or champagne to loosen up.

- Wear a dress or blouse and skirt, bra, panties, garter belt, and stockings (or thigh-highs). If you have body issues, wear a big silk shirt. Remove your bra or simply lift your breasts out of the bra, leaving it on for support—all without removing the big shirt that you will leave seductively open.

- Dim the lights.

- Put ben wa, or Oriental love balls, into your vagina, to stimulate you while you dance.

The Strip

- Take your time in getting down to the basics.

- Sit on the floor to remove stockings, arching one leg up and out, then back into your body—like a fancy sitting-down kick—before pulling off the stocking. Repeat with the other leg.

- Slip the shoes back on.

(continued on next page)

- Turn your back to him and teasingly pull down your panties. Let him see what you're doing from the rear—or the side.

- Finish the job right in front of his face. No man notices cellulite on your thighs when you put your pussy in his face.

....

 DAY 48: SEX ED SATURDAY

Arab Sex #4: Ejaculatory Control

Take the Art of Brinksmanship (page 57) a little further. Learn how to control, or at least more strongly influence, your ejaculation timing. The techniques aren't difficult, but they do require practice.

Muscle Control
- Practice squeezing and releasing the sphincter muscle (the one you use to eliminate body waste) to make it stronger.

- Strengthen your PC muscle (the one that controls the stop and start of urination) by doing Kegels.

- Use those stronger muscles to slow down intercourse. When you feel ejaculation is imminent, stop thrusting, squeeze your sphincter, and flex your PC several times.

The Three-Finger Draw
This works for some men, but not others. (It may induce rather than inhibit ejaculation. Try and see.) Using the three longest fingers of one hand, cup the area of your perineum. Press lightly.

....

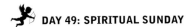

The Legend of the Yoni

Yoni is a Sanskrit word that can mean source, origin, womb, or vulva—a lot of meanings for one small word. In Hindu mythology, the goddess Shakti embodies the divine feminine energy, centered in the vulva, the yoni. She is Shiva's primary consort. Worship of her is worship of the yoni. Like Shiva, who is inseparable from his penis/lingam, she *is* her yoni/vulva.

In one myth, her body was cut to pieces—and her yoni fell to earth at Manobhavaguha Cave at Mount Nila, a cave protecting a yoni-shaped cleft, a place that is still held sacred today and is known as Kamakhya Pitha.

Although phallic worship has been studied extensively worldwide, vulva worship has not. But we can trace yoni worship throughout Hindu culture. You can find some of the most impressive monuments to the yoni in Kerala, India. Devotees still leave fruits, nuts, seeds, shells, and flowers to honor the goddess.

Worship at your pussy altar today (see page 67). Bring fresh flowers. Light the candles. Burn the incense. Let him fall to his knees and worship the vulva in the way most pleasing to her.

. . . .

Double Entendres and Coffee

Some double entendres are cringe-inducing while others sound brilliant. Don't try to be cute or smarmy or even use double-meaning words if they aren't a comfortable fit. The trick is to say something that your partner will find sexy in a very personal way—but will go right over the kids' heads.

Some ideas:

- Make a reference to the first place you had sex.

- Say, "I remember the last time you wore that blouse"—if you hurriedly took it off her.

- Say, "You have so much strength in your toes"—if he gets up on his toes in the missionary position.

- Say, "Um, that fragrance always makes me think of Paris" (or wherever you've had a romantic getaway).

- Say, "I love when you're clean-shaven"—as you stroke his face (the day after he shaved his pubic hair for you).

....

The Naked Chef

Pick a recipe from *InterCourses: An Aphrodisiac Cookbook* and cook for her in the nude, covered only by a manly apron. Select something that will give you about ten minutes of free time before serving. (I love the capellini with rosemary.) Ask her to take off her panties and put them in your apron pocket. Sit her on the kitchen counter or a high stool, pour her a glass of wine, and let her enjoy the sensual mélange of cooking smells and glimpses of your body. As the meal progresses, feed her samples with one hand while you slide your other hand up her skirt, caress her thighs, and stroke her labia.

With the meal and her pussy well in hand, take off your apron.

Holding your penis in one hand, use the head to stroke her clitoris as you are kissing her mouth.

Insert just the head into her vagina and stroke her clitoris as you take shallow strokes.

Pull out and rub the head around her clitoris as you put two fingers in her vagina.

Put the head back inside her. Keep playing with her clitoris.

As she gets more and more excited, take deeper strokes—but don't take your fingers away from her clit until you feel her orgasm building beneath your fingertips. Then drive it home.

. . . .

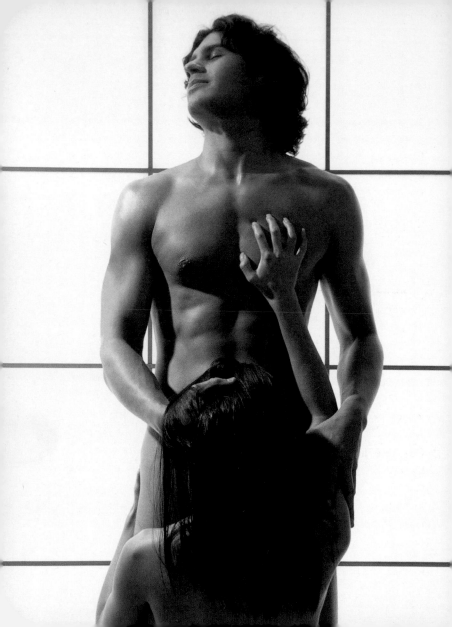

The "Cum Shake," His

Some women say they don't like the taste of their man's semen. I've never had this problem. If I like the way a man smells and tastes when I kiss him, I always like the taste of his cum. But it's true that alcohol, recreational drugs, nicotine, and the chemicals in fast food can adversely affect the taste of his spunk.

If this is an issue in your relationship, whip out the blender and create a "cum shake" using any of the following ingredients in combination:

Pineapple	Parsley
Mango	Wheatgrass
Papaya	Celery
Melons	Cardamom
Grapes	Peppermint
Apples	Lemon

Give the shake twelve to twenty-four hours to make it through your testes. And get in the habit of drinking lots of water to flush out the other stuff unless you are wiling to live on cum shakes.

············

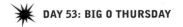 **DAY 53: BIG O THURSDAY**

The fMRI Orgasm

At Rutgers University, Dr. Barry Komisaruk, author of *The Science of Orgasm*, and his team of neuroscience researchers are studying women's orgasms with fMRI (functional magnetic resonance imaging) machines. Some women come by clitoral stimulation, others through stimulating their G-spots with a dildo, and still others through multiple forms of stimulation. A few women can "think off"—achieve a "no hands" orgasm through fantasy (and perhaps PC flexing?) alone. Women with spinal cord injuries and no feeling below the waist have orgasms, achieved through what Komisaruk describes as a "new pathway," bypassing the spine completely. This orgasm takes a detour on the vast vagus nerve network. The vagus nerves wander throughout the body— like vagabonds—and go straight to the brain.

All these orgasms look the same in the brain, which does not differentiate between "clitoral," "thinking off," or blended orgasms or any other type of orgasm. An orgasm is an orgasm in the brain, where the real sex magic happens. That is science.

If you can't afford an fMRI machine in your bedroom, go online and find graphics of your brain on orgasm. Then go to photobucket.com (the source for most of the photos illustrating SexyPrime posts) and check out the electric photographs. Now imagine your brain on orgasm—and draw it in neon markers for your lover.

....

Create a Toy Box

Go shopping tonight. Buy a sturdy storage box for your sex toys, including room for the ones you want to purchase. Stores like Target and Bed Bath & Beyond and others sell boxes in a variety of sizes and shapes, some decorative, some plain. You can use it as is, or get creative with fabric and sparkles. (If you have kids at home, you may want to protect your privacy with a box that locks.)

Put your toys inside your new box and make a wish list for future purchases. Some ideas:

- Vibrators, in a variety of sizes and styles
- Dildos
- Bondage tape/handcuffs
- Floggers
- Lubes
- Body paints
- Flavored gels

- Scented oils
- Honey dust
- Costumes
- Masks
- Paddles
- Feathers
- DVDs
- Butt plugs

. . . .

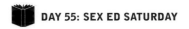

The 2,000-Year-Old BJ Position

An ancient Greece gymnasts received fellatio from skilled courtesans while in the shoulder-stand position with his genitals over her face. And she serviced him with her mouth alone, no hands. Supposedly, the tension in his thighs made his cock and balls throb.

In the modern adaptation, he lies on his back with his legs spread open in a V, feet against the headboard or wall. She straddles his chest. Yes, his cock and balls do swing free, but she uses her hands.

1. Grasp the base of his penis in one hand. You can take him straight into your mouth or at an angle.

2. With the other hand, alternate playing with his balls and lightly scratching your fingernails up and down his inner thighs.

3. Take as much of the shaft into your mouth as you comfortably can. Work it fast as you suck, swirling your tongue around the head and corona on the upstroke.

4. If he likes a finger in his anus, add that element to your hand play.

5. Position your body so that he will ejaculate straight down your throat.

············

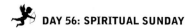 **DAY 56: SPIRITUAL SUNDAY**

Kundalini #1: Freeing the Energy

Kundalini is sexual energy. Imagine it as a fiery coil of energy located at the base of your spine—or as the coiled snake often used to illustrate it.

You will learn how to free your kundalini energy, make it rise throughout your body, and connect with your partner's rising kundalini energy. That may sound a little abstract—or too "New Age-y"—for some readers, but trust me; the energy is real. And you *can* tap into it to create more passion in your sex life.

1. Either stand with your legs comfortably apart or sit with your legs loosely folded in front of you.

2. Breathe deeply. On the inhalation, imagine that you are loosening the coils of the energy snake and enticing it upward.

3. Now light a fire under the snake to make it move faster. Imagine you are breathing hot air in through your genitals and out your nose.

4. The snake is awake.

....

Back-to-Back Snuggle

Many couples like to sleep back to back. Indulge in a face-to-face full-body caress before you roll over to your respective positions. Finally, rub butts before you fall asleep.

In the morning, spend those last few delicious moments before you have to get up pressing your backs against one another. Intertwine your legs. Rub butts again.

The back-to-back is a playful yet sensual snuggle.

....

The Vibe/Tongue/G-Spot Triple Play Quickie, Hers

This works as an oral quickie for her alone—or as intense foreplay before an intercourse quickie. Use a finger vibe. It's small, discrete, and not distracting, and it slips onto your fingertip.

Follow the track of your tongue, circling her clitoris with the finger vibe.
Suck or lick her clitoris, running the vibe along the sides.
Stimulate her labia with it.
Using two fingers, stroke her G-spot as you continue cunnilingus moves, enhanced by your vibrating finger.

....

The Historical BJ #2: The Duchess of Windsor's Butterfly Throat

The compelling love story of the Duke and Duchess of Windsor continues to fascinate women of all ages. Why? King Edward gave up the English throne for this American divorcee, who wasn't particularly attractive. Obviously, she had something—and that something was, according to reliable sources, *sex*.

She studied sex techniques in the East before she met Edward. Her specialty was said to be the ability to make both her vagina and her throat quiver, like the beating of a butterfly's wings. Yes, she not only performed a deep throat maneuver, but she also made it flutter. Here's the easier version:

1. Practice "fluttering" your throat by making an *ah-ah-ah-ah* sound deep in your throat.

2. Vibrate the sound.

3. Keep practicing.

4. When you can comfortably vibrate your throat, do it while you are giving him a BJ. Even if you can't deep throat him at the same time, the fluttery move will vibrate your mouth and tongue—and his cock.

. . . .

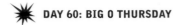 **DAY 60: BIG O THURSDAY**

The Secret Orgasm Mind-Set, Hers

I call the secret orgasm mind-set "claiming pleasure." The idea that women who reach orgasm easily *have made up their minds* to claim their pleasure grew out of the stories women tell me. At some point, they decide: I want it, I will take it, orgasm is mine. Often, they write about how finding their sexual pleasure changed their lives in other ways. In discovering orgasm, for example, they found their self-confidence and became more effective at work and in all their relationships. After finally asserting their needs and desires to longtime partners, they knocked down the barricades and found the intimacy they craved. Or they realized they would never find it there but they did have the courage to move on. No woman is truly empowered unless she is sexually empowered.

"I had my first orgasm—and it not only rocked my body, it changed my world," a twenty-eight-year-old woman wrote. "I lost my virginity and faked my first orgasm when I was fifteen. I knew how to fake an orgasm from watching movies, not even porn. It didn't occur to me that the women probably had to fake because they weren't getting clitoral stimulation. I thought she was supposed to come from what her lover did to her, especially intercourse. I didn't have skilled lovers; I was playing with boys and whatever they did to me, oral or manual, wasn't enough."

If you don't have as many orgasms as you would like to have, then change your mind-set. Declare that, from this day forward, you will claim your pleasure. He doesn't have to give it to you because you can take it for yourself—and paradoxically, that makes the gift all the sweeter when he does give it.

. . . .

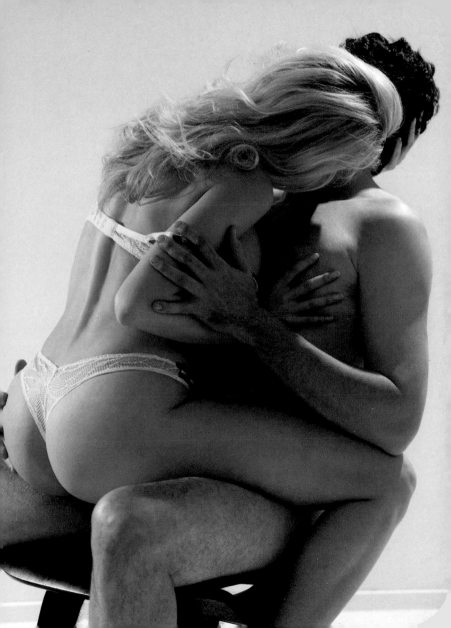

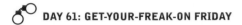 **DAY 61: GET-YOUR-FREAK-ON FRIDAY**

Anal Orgasm, His

You found your G-spot on page 66. Stimulating that spot either exter-
nally by pressing the perineum or internally by a finger inserted into the
anus is very arousing for many men. Some men can have an orgasm via
G-spot stimulation. Strictly speaking, it's an anal orgasm.

There are three ways to make it happen.

Manual
She strokes his G-spot with a well-lubricated finger or two or a slender
anal vibe.

Oral
Shower or bathe together first. He gets down on all fours on the bed—
the same position she assumes for rear-entry intercourse. From behind,
she licks his anus in broad strokes, then penetrates him with the tip of
her tongue. (For protection against bacteria, use a sheet of plastic wrap.)

Intercourse
See Strap-On Thrusting Techniques, page 295.

....

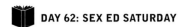

Puritan Sex #1:
Repressed but Dirty, Clothes On

We've all read *The Scarlet Letter*, Nathaniel Hawthorne's novel of Puritan sexual repression, adultery, and punishment. Sex before marriage was so common among the uptight Puritans, however, that one study of old family bibles found that more than half first babies were born seven months after their parents married. In their own way, our national ancestors encouraged premarital sex. Young unwed couples were allowed to sleep over, separated by a bundling board, a narrow board down the center of the bed. Imagine running that past today's parents of teens.

Steep yourself in cultural repression—and do it like the Puritans tonight. Don't take your clothes off.

Outercourse (or Dry Humping)

Make out like teenagers. Kiss and caress, touch and grab and squeeze. Breathless youthful groping is hot. But play by the rules your parents or grandparents were supposed to follow:

- He can reach inside her bra and caress her breast—but he can't remove her top and bra.

- They can fondle one another's genitals through clothes only.

- Lie, one on top of the other, and bump and grind. Hump your way to orgasms.

....

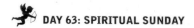

The Spiritual Orgasm: Extra-Genital

Some women and a very few men can reach orgasm by extra-genital stimulation to nipples or breasts, inner thighs, neck, ears, belly, buttocks, and even toes. Coming without genital stimulation feels like an almost spiritual experience. Most likely, it will happen after multiple orgasms achieved the old-fashioned way, through genital stimulation.

When she is blessed out—and thinks she is spent—following multiple Os, try this:

1. Caress her genitals orally and manually until she is on the verge of orgasm again.

2. Stop.

3. Shift your attention to nongenital areas.

4. Alternate from genital stimulation to nongenital until she is so aroused—and hypersensitive—that you can bring her to orgasm by sucking her nipple or running your fingers down her inner thighs.

Her orgasm will feel like it begins in the genitals (no matter where the triggering touch is) and expands throughout her entire body.

....

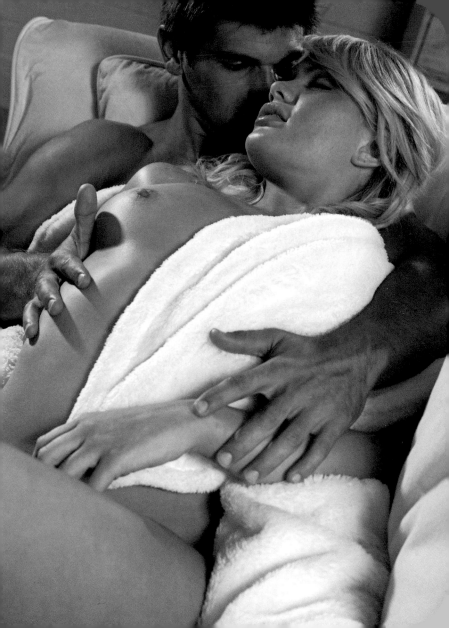

DAY 64: FLIRTATION AND FOREPLAY MONDAY

The Good-Night Feather

In real life, couples do sometimes go to bed mad. Occasionally, one may not be speaking to the other. The state of not speaking can even be mutual.

Keep a lush feather in your nightstand drawer. (I have a big fluffy black feather on a lacquered stem. Elegant.) On nights when there is a little tension in the bed between you, take out the feather.

- Lightly tickle his or her ear.

- Run the feather under his chin.

- Stroke it along his neck and up to the other ear.

- Tickle his nose—and follow that with a light kiss.

- Good night.

....

DAY 65: QUICKIE TUESDAY

The Vibrating Cock Ring Quickie

Vibrating cock rings come in a limited range of styles. It's a simple concept: a ring that slides around the cock, fits at the base, and holds a small vibe. Even a marketing strategist can't come up with too many ways of putting that package together.

Disposable cock rings are nice for singles and traveling couples, but the vibrating power is less than that of reusable cock rings, typically run by bullet vibes. Buy a nice stretchy one. The hard rings aren't very comfortable and can be harmful if worn too long.

Unless you are just doing this for him, strap on a sweetheart vibe or put on your vibrating panties.

As you are giving him oral or manual foreplay, slip the cock ring onto his erect shaft, slide it down to the base, and turn it on.

Continue to play with him—and pay attention to his balls, made exquisitely sensitive by the vibrations.

Leave his cock ring on during intercourse in whatever quickie position you choose.

....

 DAY 66: ORAL WEDNESDAY

The L-Shaped Cunnilingus Position

Women perform fellatio on our knees on the floor, between his legs in bed, either lying outstretched or kneeling, or from the side of his body or lying on our backs, sometimes with our heads hanging over the edge of the bed. Men, however, tend to perform cunnilingus mostly from the front, either kneeling between her legs or lying flat. Try it a new way: Kneel at her hip at a right angle to her body.

Changes your perspective, doesn't it? Changes her sensations, too.

(continued on next page)

Tips for making the new angle work:

- Your tongue won't naturally stray downward to lap at her labia—so make it up with your (lubed) fingers.

- Put two fingers on either side of her clit and press down lightly as you lick and suck.

- Purse your lips more loosely when you do the Velvet "No" move (page 26).

- Lean over her body so that your mouth is positioned straight over her clit. Now come straight down with the tip of your tongue and flick back and forth very lightly on the tip of her clit.

- From the same straight down position, circle the shaft with the tip of your tongue, slowly at first, then picking up speed.

....

✳ **DAY 67: BIG O THURSDAY**

Vibrating Massage with His Happy Ending

Build on the vibe power you unleashed in Tuesday's quickie! Get him naked and give him an erotic massage—with vibrator—and a happy ending. Start with a body massage. Rub his shoulders. Massage his back, thighs, and buttocks.

After that, he will probably have an erection. Straddle it but don't insert it. Lower your breasts to his body and tease his nipples by rubbing yours across his. Or take your nipples in hand and rub them across his.

In the straddle position, move down his body so that you end up kneeling between his legs. Take his testicles between your fingers and thumb gently, one at a time. Then hold a testicle in the palm of your hand and tickle it lightly with the pads of your fingers. Now the other one.

Hold the base of his penis in one hand and work your other hand in a circular fashion to the head. Use the palm of that hand to caress the head of his penis.

As if you were building a fire with his penis as the stick, use a rolling/rubbing motion, starting at the base. Roll/rub up to the head and back down to the base, keeping his penis between your palms. Start slowly. Increase speed and pressure as he gets close to orgasm.

Now surprise him by pulling out a vibrator.

Start on a low speed. Run the vibe along the shaft of his penis. Press it against the base, the scrotum, and the perineum.

Guided by his response, experiment with higher speeds and firmer pressures. But don't apply more powerful vibrators directly to his penis. Hold it against the back of your hand as your hold the shaft of his penis. Move his penis up and down with your vibrating hand.

When he is near ejaculation, lean forward so that he comes onto your breasts. To make him come quickly, insert a finger into his anus and press gently.

....

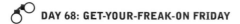 **DAY 68: GET-YOUR-FREAK-ON FRIDAY**

The Imaginary Friend Threesome

What couple hasn't at least toyed with the idea of a threesome? (Some statistics put participation as high as 25 percent and those who have fantasized at 75 percent.)

If bringing a real person into your bed isn't an option, then create an imaginary playmate. It worked when you were kids and let your imaginations run free. Why not now?

Open your toy box and take out a dildo or a penis sleeve. (Your guest needs genitals, right?)

Make a threesome partner wish list, probably not including in-laws and best friends. Brad or Angelina or Jen, fine.

Select a partner. (If he wants a woman and she wants a man, take turns.)

One person can play two roles, self and imaginary partner. Or you can just pretend he or she is there and take turns describing the action from that perspective.

Put on a threesome DVD, like Tristan Taormino's *Expert Guide to Threesomes*, which is both educational and hot.

Use those toys!

. . . .

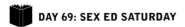 **DAY 69: SEX ED SATURDAY**

Blindfold Games

If you haven't seen the classic film *9½ Weeks* with Mickey Rourke and
Kim Basinger, rent it now. Blindfold games are designed to heighten
your other senses: taste, smell, hearing, and touch. Take turns wearing
the blindfold.

The Food Game
The blindfolded partner doesn't know what taste to expect next. You'll
be surprised at how different some things taste when you don't see them
before they enter your mouth. Without visual cues, you are operating on
taste and smell.

The Feather or the Flogger Game
Your lover doesn't know whether he will feel a gentle tickle or a light
sting across his nipples, thighs, or buttocks. Anticipation makes the skin
wake up and pay attention.

The Sexy Whispers Game
Try arousing your lover with your voice alone. Whisper sexy words—everything from erotic poems to dirty talk. Let her feel your breath in her ear,
on her neck. Pause occasionally to nibble her earlobe, then switch ears.

Blind Sex
One of you can leave the blindfold on during lovemaking or you can take
turns wearing it.

············

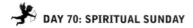 **DAY 70: SPIRITUAL SUNDAY**

Slow Sex

You have time and you want to make the sex last. He's on top and you are close to orgasm. Instead of pushing for it, you pull back and put your hands on his butt to guide him into a gentle rhythm. But you feel him losing some of his erection.

Keep it slow and keep him hard at the same time. Clench your PC muscle hard, firmly enough to hold him in place. Grab his hips or buttocks and rock him, side to side or back and forth, flexing your PC in time with the move. Ask him to play with your clit if you need that extra stimulation.

You are controlling the direction of his pelvic movements, the speed of thrusting, and the depth of penetration, and you have him where you need him. You can keep him there until you come, and he will likely regain his erection. He will probably have an orgasm, too, and it will feel to him like you are pulling the orgasm out of him in an explosive way.

············

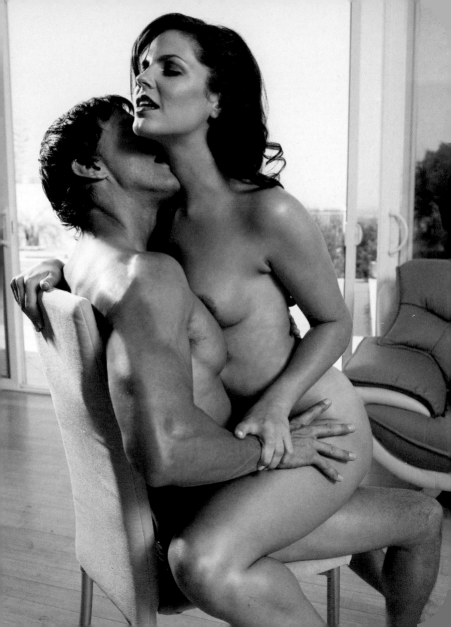

Flashing

An unexpected glimpse of genitals—even familiar ones—is surprising and sexy. Remember all the uproar over a momentary view of Janet Jackson's nipple during the 2004 Super Bowl halftime show? The key to a good flash: It has to be done on the run. Otherwise, it's an invitation to play.

His Flash

You're dressed for work, and you're leaving first. Before you go out the door, quickly and quietly unzip your pants and let her see your erection. (You'll get one just thinking about doing this.)

Her Flash

After you've kissed him good-bye, reach inside your bra, pull your breast out, and let him have a quick look, no touch. Or as you're leaving, raise your skirt and show him you're not wearing panties.

....

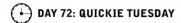

Tweaking the Standing Position

The standing intercourse position is the classic quickie pose. Don't you feel like a star on a film set whenever you assume this position? Yes, you do—because it looks so hot.

Typically, your leg is wrapped around his waist while his hands clasp your buttocks. One of you has your back against a wall for more support.

In this variation, she stands against the wall on a staircase while he stands in front of her. Putting one leg on the banister behind him, she grasps his buttocks and pulls him into her. Using her raised leg for leverage, she controls the thrusting.

....

DAY 73: ORAL WEDNESDAY

The Ring and the Seal, His

If he has a large penis or thrusts more vigorously into your mouth than you like, then I've got a move for you. Created by Lou Paget (a sister sexpert), the Ring and the Seal both elongates your mouth—making him feel like he's going deeper—and gives you better control over how much and how fast you take his penis into your mouth. I've taught this simple move to women who tell me it changed their attitude about fellatio in the most positive way.

Form the Ring and Seal by making a circle with the fingers and thumb of one hand. Put the ring around your mouth. Your hand stays sealed, attached to your mouth, as you perform fellatio.

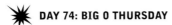

DAY 74: BIG O THURSDAY

Playing Her Hot Spots

Men and women both have "hot spots," places extremely sensitive to touch, oral and manual. You know where most are, but you may not be hitting them effectively in foreplay, oral sex, and intercourse.

The C-Spot

Her clitoris. The small pink organ, located at the point where the inner labia join at the top of the vaginal opening, also includes the clitoral hood, interior parts, and a network of nerve endings. Don't neglect the area surrounding the pink shaft. Stroke it with fingers while you're tonguing the shaft.

The G-Spot

That small mass of rough tissue about a third of the way up the front vaginal wall may or may not exist in your lover. If it does, stroke it with your finger or a G-spot vibe while you are giving her cunnilingus.

The AFE Zone

The anterior fornix erotic (AFE) zone is a small patch of skin closer to the cervix than the G-spot is. Stroking the AFE zone makes most women lubricate immediately. Do that before intercourse.

The U-Spot

The tiny area of tissue above the opening of the urethra and right below the clitoris is a pleasure point for many women. If her clitoris is too sensitive for touch immediately after her first orgasm, move your tongue here.

Individual Hot Spots

Most women have other spots. Breasts and nipples, neck and ears, backs of knees, hollow of the throat, that little hollow at the base of her back, and toes are all potential hot spots. Explore with fingers and tongue.

....

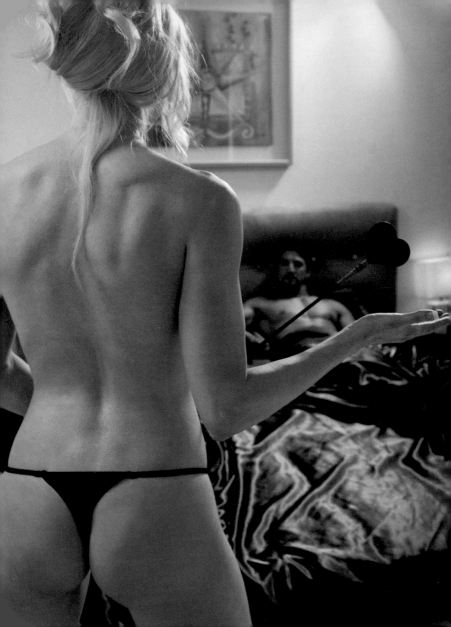

DAY 75: GET-YOUR-FREAK-ON FRIDAY

Flogger Strokes

The floggers sold in sex toy shops and online have soft suede lashes. But if you use one with enough force, you can leave a mark. That's a little too freaky for most people. Try out the flogger on your own flesh before you use it on your partner. How does it feel on the sensitive skin of *your* inner thighs?

Here are some tips for getting the most out of your flogger:

- Start with a stroke so light that it feels like blades of grass moving in the wind.

- Don't keep flogging the same spot. Move it around.

- Pick up the intensity slightly.

- Be guided by your lover's responses as you use a firmer stroke.

- Land the firmest strokes on the fleshiest parts of the buttocks.

....

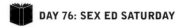 **DAY 76: SEX ED SATURDAY**

Looking in Her Mirror

Women are encouraged to look at their genitals in a mirror. (Remember the *Sex and the City* episode where Samantha encouraged Charlotte to check herself out?) Men can learn something by looking in her mirror, too. Even when you're right on top of her genitals, you're often not getting a good look. So use a hand mirror.

After she's showered or bathed, gently part her labia with lubed fingers. Notice how the sets of lips come together.

Gently pull back the clitoral hood, exposing the shaft.

Hold the mirror at the opening of her vagina as she holds her lips open and take a little peek inside.

....

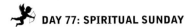 **DAY 77: SPIRITUAL SUNDAY**

Kundalini #2:
Connecting Your Energies

You learned how to awaken and free the coiled snake of your individual sexual energies on page 83. Now you will connect the snakes. The ancient Egyptians believed they did this in religious rituals we might describe as orgies. Fueled by wine and drugs, they danced their energies—which they depicted as cobras—up into their genitals and, through sexual contact, all the way up their bodies into their heads.

1. Sit with legs loosely folded in front of your bodies, across from one another on the floor or bed.

2. Take deep breaths. Synchronize your breathing so that you are inhaling and exhaling together. Imagine the coiled kundalini energies coming to life and moving toward your genitals.

3. Make body contact. Touch feet, hold hands, or entwine your lower legs, whatever is comfortable.

4. Imagine that you are breathing separate circles of fire, in through your genitals, out through your mouths.

5. The circles grow bigger. They touch one another and then overlap. Do you feel your kundalini energy infusing your genitals and reaching toward your lover's?

6. Let the snakes mate.

············

👁 **DAY 78: FLIRTATION AND FOREPLAY MONDAY**

The Stranger at the Dinner Table

You could pretend to be strangers meeting for an Internet-arranged dinner at a restaurant, but save your entertainment money for tomorrow night. Tonight, pretend you don't know everything about each other. (Really, you don't.) Ask new questions. Listen to answers. Getting to know someone is seductive.

Conversation Starters

- What sexual secret did you keep from your parents and siblings when you were thirteen?

- Tell me what you did after your first kiss.

- How did you know you were in love for the first time?

- What did it feel like to touch a girl's breast or pussy or a boy's penis for the first time?

- Who was your first crush?

- What was the best time you ever had masturbating?

....

🕐 DAY 79: QUICKIE TUESDAY

The Bar "Hookup"

This game is played two ways. The couple pretends to be strangers and "meet" at a bar after work. They attract a lot of attention by flirting openly, even kissing passionately. In one scenario, they go to the restroom together and have a quickie; in the other, they go home together (where they have their quickie).

Play It a New Way

Take it further publicly than you ever have, even if you do it in a back booth. For example:

- Rest her hand in his lap—over the bulge in his trousers.

- Let his hand slide up her thigh beneath her skirt—and disappear.

- Keep up the hand play as you drink and talk—with his other hand grazing her breast and hers playing inside his shirt buttons.

- Entwine your legs. Rub calves and thighs.

- He can stand behind her barstool and kiss her neck while briefly caressing her breasts (through her blouse).

- She can stand behind his barstool and put her arms around him, trailing them down his chest and into his lap.

- *Now* you can move to the kissing.

....

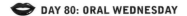

Head Games #2: The Deep Suck, His

Some men say their erections grow stronger with this kind of sucking. You may need a little practice to pull it off, but will he find that bothersome? I don't think so.

Gradually suck the full length of his penis (or as much as you can) into your mouth—the slower the better. Move your tongue around the shaft as you're sucking in.

Once you have him in, pull in the sides of your cheeks to create suction. Relax the back of your throat. Give his penis several hard sucks.

Open your mouth to release the suction.

When you close your mouth again, pull in the sides of your cheeks again before sucking.

Bonus points: If you can, tease the corona with the tip of your tongue while you're sucking.

Short-Circuiting the Gag Reflex

• Some women say they won't gag if his penis doesn't touch the insides of their cheeks.

• Others take frequent swallows.

• Still others flatten their tongue against his penis when they feel like gagging.

....

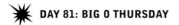 **DAY 81: BIG O THURSDAY**

Playing His Hot Spots

It's his turn. Tonight, play his hot spots.

The H-Spot
Head of the penis. Don't neglect the corona when you swirl and suck it.

The F-Spot
Strum this loose section of skin on the underside of the penis where the head meets the shaft it with the tip of your tongue. Suck it gently.

The R Area
The raphe area is the visible line along the center of the scrotum. It may be the most neglected spot on a man's body. Lick it slowly up and down. Then flick your tongue rapidly back and forth up the raphe, then down again.

The P Zone
The perineum zone is an area an inch or so in size, between the base of the anus and the scrotum. Though sadly overlooked, this is the second most important hot spot for some men. Experiment with stroking and gently pushing against the perineum.

The G-Spot
This is inside the body, behind the perineum. Insert a well-lubed finger into his anus and stroke it. (See page 66 for more on how to locate it.)

. . . .

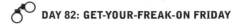 **DAY 82: GET-YOUR-FREAK-ON FRIDAY**

The Freak Talk

Have you been harboring a secret desire for something a little "freaky" but you're embarrassed or nervous to tell your partner? Each write a sex scenario about something you haven't done together. Read your stories out loud. Ask one another basic questions, such as:

"Is this something you would like to do with me?"
"How do you see it working out?"
"Can I make some adjustments?"
"What if I change my mind about doing it midway through?"

Negotiate the terms this way, without having a serious "freak-on" talk.

To get you started, read this from a SexyPrime reader, writing to his lover:

What She Should Do to My Cock:

Slide on a cock ring. Gentle kisses up and down the shaft with a wet, caressing tongue, paying special attention to the bottom of the head. Light feathery touches/tickles/scratches to a tight sac. Continue this until the head is engorged and leaking precum—and my cock is straining against the ring. Lightly squeeze and scratch my balls.

Continue until I'm out of my mind, then take the entire shaft into her mouth slowly and deliberately. Very slow until the pressure is unbearable. Even after reflexive attempts at thrusting, continue the unbearably slow, deliberate, hot engulfing until it explodes, in her mouth or on her breasts.

The key word is unbearable. Make me beg for release.

....

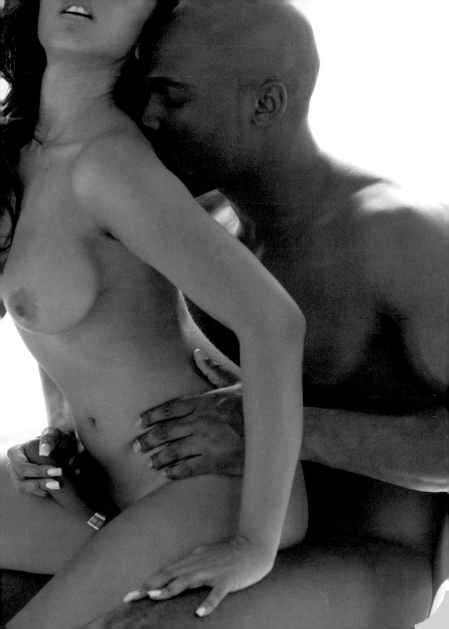

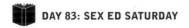 **DAY 83: SEX ED SATURDAY**

Arab Sex #5: The Seducer Position

The seducer, the man, is in charge here. Like the other Arabian inter-course positions, the Seducer is designed to give him maximum control and her maximum pleasure. Who can argue with that?

1. She lies on her back with her legs open.

2. He sits on his folded legs between her legs.

3. Separating her thighs to accommodate the width of his torso, he lifts up her buttocks and places her legs under his arms.

4. With her legs secured, he puts his arms under her waist and pulls her onto his penis.

5. He guides the thrusting by pushing her back and forth.

6. If the position is difficult for her to maintain, she can place her hands on his shoulders or forearms for support. (And she can wear a sweetheart vibe to make her orgasm more certain.)

············

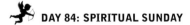 **DAY 84: SPIRITUAL SUNDAY**

Telling Secrets, Confessing Desires

Maybe you have never told her how you felt after the first time you made love to each other. Or that at one time you lost interest in him—but thrillingly got it back. Again, writing is easier than saying.

This comes from another SexyPrime reader describing a memorable first orgasmic experience with the cougar he now loves:

I didn't think I wanted her—or she me. She isn't beautiful, but sexy in a carnal way, a smart cougar who takes the measure of your cock by looking into your eyes.

The foreplay was speeded up and she was the one on the fast track. Removing only her black skirt and black lace panties, she laid back on the bed, white shirt open, black lace bra exposed. Missionary position. I crawled obediently between her great legs. She wrapped one around my waist and rested the calf of the other on my shoulder, one red stiletto close enough to do some harm.

I began thrusting inside her. She fingered her clit, eyes closed or looking past mine. I thrust faster and harder. Her first orgasm bubbled up beneath her fingertips. I felt it move into her pussy. She looked into my eyes then.

"I want you," she said. I wanted her, too. I leaned over to kiss her. She pulled that leg around my neck and held me. When she closed her eyes, I said, "Damn it, look at me."

She came again, eyes looking inside me. Now she was in my head and I in hers. My orgasm built deep inside my balls; and I ached for those spasms. I fucked her hard and fast and she was with me. I felt such intense release that tears sprang to my eyes. She licked them as she flexed her pussy around my still quivering cock.

I felt powerful until she grazed me with her heel. It was her game. It didn't matter.

. . . .

DAY 85: FLIRTATION AND FOREPLAY MONDAY

Panties in the Pocket

When you hand a man your panties on your way out the door, you've captured his imagination. He will think about you after you've gone— and perhaps wonder if anyone will get a glimpse of your naked pussy if you cross your legs on the train. It's a really effective move if one or the other of you is going out of town for the night or will be out very late at a business or social event.

Make sure he sees you put on panties. They'll pick up a bit of your scent as you wear them through breakfast. Then casually step out of them, hand them to him, and say, "Keep my panties in your pocket for me."

....

The Fusion Tantra Counter Quickie

The Tantra celebrated in the West focuses on emotional and spiritual connection over technique, and devotees insist it takes time. Who has time? I created Fusion Tantra to combine the sex techniques of the East with the goal-oriented sex philosophy of the West. Fusion Tantra speeds arousal and intensifies orgasm. I hope you will read my book *The New Tantra: Simple and Sexy*. Meanwhile, it's Quickie Tuesday and you need to take advantage of it. This one is simple—and effective.

1. He sits on the kitchen counter.

2. She sits down on his penis.

3. Leaning forward, she lifts herself three-quarters of the way up his penis, putting her hands on his shoulders for balance.

4. She moves her pelvis to the right, pushing herself down at the same time.

5. She pulls back up and moves her pelvis to the left, again pushing herself down at the same time.

6. Go back and forth like this for as long as you both want.

....

The Historical BJ #3:
Cleopatra's Cobra Blow Job

Cleopatra conquered Caesar and Anthony, two of Rome's great leaders. Clearly, she was good in bed. Often pictured in bas relief with a snake (asp or cobra) held to her smiling lips, she was also, or so historians have assumed, a skilled oral lover. She is sometimes referred to as "the great swallower" or "she of the wide mouth" and rumored to have performed her specialty on men at royal galas.

This is how she may have done it:

Sometimes a queen wants to kneel before her favorite cock, take it into her hands and mouth, feel it come to vibrant life, and bring it extreme pleasure. On such a night when she feels her erotic power coursing through her, she sits him in a chair . . .

- Put a cushion on the floor between his open legs. Kneel. From this position you can come straight down on his head with your mouth—not the most effective position for deep throating but a very good position for stimulating the head and corona—or in this case, the head of the cobra.

- Work your hand magic loosely up his shaft to maintain his erection while you focus most of the oral attention on his head.

- Repeatedly circle the head with your wet tongue. Give it light sucks, with your lips covering the corona between swirls.

- Follow the ridge of the corona with the tip of your tongue. Pick up the movement. Create a whirling pace.

- Sway lightly back and forth like a snake charmer as you swirl and suck the head and whirl around his corona.

- Let his cum dribble out the sides of your mouth. Look into his eyes as you rub his cum into your nipples.

....

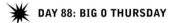 **DAY 88: BIG O THURSDAY**

The New Woman on Top #2:
The Ultimate Lap Dance

This one looks as good to him as it feels to you. Imagine giving him a lap dance as you're riding his penis. The sensual undulations of your torso will give him a real visual treat. The bonus: a bigger orgasm for you.

These two simple moves vary the up-and-down intercourse motion:

- Lean slightly forward and push your pubis slightly back on the downward move (stimulating your clitoris with the shaft).

- Lean slightly backward and push your pubis slightly forward on the upward movement (stimulating your G-spot with the head of the penis).

Put the moves together in a continuous motion that looks like you are dancing seductively on his penis. Use your hands—caress your breasts, tweak your nipples, and play with your clitoris.

....

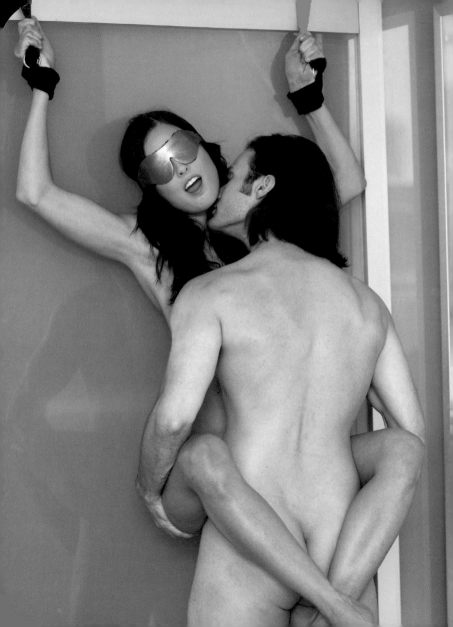

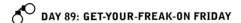 **DAY 89: GET-YOUR-FREAK-ON FRIDAY**

BDSM Vanilla: The Roles and the Rules

The vast majority of us are "vanilla" people—into straight sex with light kinky variations. Few couples live in DS (dominant/submissive) or BDSM (bondage, discipline, sadomasochistic) relationships. How does a vanilla couple put a little spice into their sexual repertoire? Serious BDSM players live by this rule: safe, sane, and consensual. Amateurs can misinterpret a partner's fantasy and deliver a hard spanking, for example, when a softer one is really desired. They might tie a partner too tightly or fail to see that a gag is causing a panic attack.

A Quickie Guide to Light Kink

- There are two basic roles: dominant and submissive. Switch them around.

- Buy your toys at a store such as Babeland (or online at Babeland. com), where you can get instructions on using them safely. Test equipment on yourself before using it on your partner. How does that gag feel? Those handcuffs? That belt whacked across your thighs?

- Adopt a safe word or phrase like the players use. That word shouldn't be "no" because saying "oh, no, no" when you mean "oh, yes, yes" is part of the game. Choose something like "red" or "peanut butter," which you both acknowledge means STOP.

- If you try something to please your partner and don't like it, you don't have to do it again. (Partner, don't nag or whine.) Realize that fantasies are not wishes meant to be acted upon. Interpreting them takes some skill. Work it out together.

. . . .

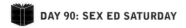 **DAY 90: SEX ED SATURDAY**

Chinese Sex #1: Pillow Books

The oldest surviving sex manual was written by Huang Ti, the Yellow Emperor, in about 2500 BCE. Writing in a question-and-answer format, the emperor asked the goddess Wise Maiden how to seduce and satisfy a woman. That book was the precursor of the Taoist pillow books, small sex instruction manuals, each on a specific topic with explicit illustrations.

Create your own pillow books.

1. Buy attractive journals with blank paper and label them, for example, Fellatio, Cunnilingus, Intercourse Positions, etc.

2. Cut out erotic photos and drawings from magazines or old books and paste them into your pillow books.

3. Copy your favorite sex technique recipes from my books onto the pages.

4. Add your notes about how you adapted techniques.

5. Include erotic poems, pressed flowers, cards, and mementos.

....

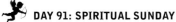 **DAY 91: SPIRITUAL SUNDAY**

Communicating with His Cock

You're both relaxing in bed. This is the perfect time to throw off the sheets and commune with his cock. Slide down your man's body, take his cock in your hands, and look at it, really look.

- What shape is it? Thin and long? Short and thick? Slightly curved?

Have you thought what the cock might want based on its shape and size? You can take a thin, short one up your ass. You can use a curve to get G-spot stimulation.

- How hard does it usually get?

Some penises, especially exceptionally large ones, do not ever get very hard. Others lose some of their erectile strength with age. Other penises will achieve youthful erections into their forties, fifties, and beyond. If he's on the softer side, build more hand jobs and blow jobs into your repertoire. Keep your PC muscle in good working order and adapt positions, such as wrapping your legs around his waist in missionary.

- Do you recognize the stages of his arousal pattern?

There's more to a penis than erection and post-ejaculation. As he approaches orgasm, his heart rate, breathing, and blood pressure reach their peaks and he is as hard as he is going to get. His thrusting reaches a peak.

- Would you like to say anything to his penis while you're down there?

Dr. Sonia Borg, creator of the Penis Whisperer BJ, says: "Put your mouth around his clothed penis and make the humming sound coming from deep in your throat. This will send vibrations up and down his spine and give him something too yummy to think about for the next few minutes."

I adore Sonia's joyous approach to sex, and it makes me want to say "I love you" to my favorite cock.

....

Paint Her Toenails

One of the sexiest (and savviest) women I ever knew began a relationship with the man she would later marry by having him paint her toenails. They were both staying at a hotel in Beverly Hills and met poolside. He told her she had pretty feet. She said, "I'll meet you back here tomorrow with polish. You can paint my toes."

Fortunately, he didn't turn out to be a foot fetishist.

Get a pedicure or at least remove old polish and use a pumice stone on the rough patches. Put your nice smooth feet in his lap while you're watching TV together. Casually ask him, "Would you mind painting my toenails?"

....

DAY 93: QUICKIE TUESDAY

Quickie Foreplay Phone Sex/Texting

Mental foreplay generally precedes a good quickie. He keeps thinking about the way she looked shaking her breasts into her bra that morning. She finds herself daydreaming about the way he held her a few beats longer than usual as he kissed her good-bye. Sometimes the mental foreplay needs a technology boost.

Mid-morning, leave a suggestive voice mail in your huskiest voice.

At lunchtime, send a quick text, such as, "Wish I were eating u."

Mid-afternoon, connect briefly on the phone. Ask him to put his hand on his cock. Ask her to slide her hand inside her panties.

Before you leave work, send one more voice mail, describing how he or she looks in orgasm.

. . . .

DAY 94: ORAL WEDNESDAY

The Swallow, His

Men feel totally accepted and loved when you swallow, and it's not that difficult. Control the depth of penetration by using the Ring and the Seal (page 102). Position yourself so that his ejaculate will shoot straight down your throat.

These are the two easiest swallowing positions:

(continued on next page)

1. Lie on your back with your head off the edge of the bed. Your mouth and throat will form a smooth line in this position. Have him straddle your face for the elegant finish to a perfect BJ.

2. He stands while you kneel in front of him. Adjust your position so your chin is raised, elongating your throat.

If you don't want to swallow, make him come when you want him to come. Recognize the subtle signs that he is close to the point of ejaculation. Men are creatures of orgasmic habit. He may hold his breath or breathe with more intensity, make a certain sound—a grunt, a cry, an exclamation—or go silent. And his balls *will* rise closer to his body.

Now that you know his moment, you can trigger it by stimulating his G-spot with your thumb or finger pressed against his perineum, the space between his anus and the base of his testicles, or by inserting a well-lubed finger inside his anus to stimulate the G-spot from inside, but only if he is comfortable with having that done.

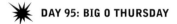

DAY 95: BIG O THURSDAY

The New Missionary #1: Legs Closed

This variation on the classic, like the Reverse Cowgirl, flips everything. He's still on top but she is lying on her stomach. It's a good change-up position, nice for when she's tired or he wants to slow down, or they're not feeling strongly connected to one another. "Intimacy" is a fluctuating state that sometimes works better without face-to-face contact.

1. She lies face down on her stomach, with her legs straight and closed.

2. Balancing his weight on his arms, he lies on top of her, one leg on either side of her, keeping his legs straight and enclosing her legs between them.

3. She squeezes her thighs on his penis as he thrusts into her.

The sensations are new and interesting. She can also flex her PC muscle, pulling him into her and pushing him out.

. . . .

 DAY 96: GET-YOUR-FREAK-ON FRIDAY

Role-Playing: Upstairs/Downstairs Sex

Play like the naughty Victorian English. The master lived upstairs, the maid downstairs. Neither displayed a flicker of impropriety in public.

The Setting
Turn your bedroom into a masculine boudoir by putting scarves over the lights, removing feminine touches, bringing a straight-backed chair into the room, and generally creating an aura of rich manliness.

The Preliminary Action
She wears a little maid's uniform—a short black skirt and blouse or dress with a white apron works, with high heels but without panties and no stockings (because she can't afford them). She uses her feather duster while he sits in his chair, watching her. He directs her to bend over to pick up something. When she does, he slaps her bare ass.

(continued on next page)

The Sex

He follows her around the room as she dusts. When she leans forward, he encircles her waist, reaches up, and squeezes a breast. As the foreplay continues, he removes her clothes until she is down to heels and bra.

When she climbs onto the bed to polish the headboard, he commands her to get down on all fours. Coming from behind, he performs cunnilingus on her until she is dripping wet and panting. He enters her and thrusts vigorously. Although they don't kiss or cuddle or express tenderness, he may bite her neck or nibble her ears.

....

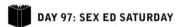 **DAY 97: SEX ED SATURDAY**

Chinese Sex #2:
Restrained Exploration

Thirty-five hundred years before the sexual revolution of the 1960s and '70s, the Chinese were liberated. They had a very sophisticated sexual philosophy that valued skill and exploration within the spiritual structure of Taoism. A religious and philosophical movement, Taoism was more enlightened than the Paganism practiced by western Europeans at the time.

According to Taoist belief, everything in life has an equal and opposite reaction. Balance is prized, especially in the yang, male energy, and the yin, female energy. You don't have to become a Taoist to find elements in the belief system that will enrich your sex life.

The components of this balanced approach to sexual exploration are:

Highly Erotic Sex
Visual sexual materials are not pornographic. They are both arousing and educational, part of foreplay and private study. Build your own collection of erotica, books, art, and quality DVDs that are arousing and aesthetically pleasing.

Athletic Positions
Although the intercourse positions are not as contorted as Kama Sutra poses, they are athletic. Work out or take a yoga class together to stay in shape for great sex, while getting in touch with your own body. The positions can also be adapted for twenty-first-century lovers.

Poetic Sex
The Taoist soul is poetic. Sexual positions are elegant in their athleticism, expressive of ecstasy. Keep a book of erotic poems on your night table and read them aloud to one another occasionally.

Belief in the Essential Nature of Sex
The belief that sex is essential to the well-being of body, mind, and soul is the cornerstone of Taoism. Modern research supports that conclusion. Regular satisfying sex has many health benefits.

．．．．．．．．．．．．

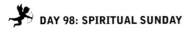 **DAY 98: SPIRITUAL SUNDAY**

Communicating with Her Pussy

In the Chinese Tang dynasty, Empress Wu Huo (who ruled 683–705 CE) insisted that all visiting male dignitaries pay her homage by performing

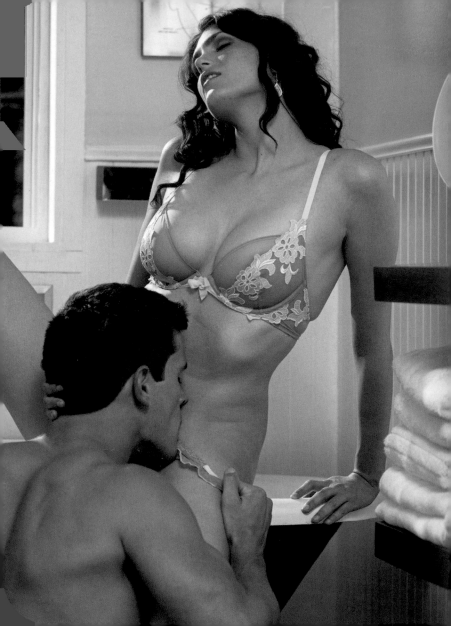

oral sex on her. Did they spend a few minutes in worship of her vulva? When I ran the Vulva Surveys on SexyPrime, I discovered that many of my male readers are modern vulva worshippers.

From a devotee:

I've gone down on almost every woman I've gone to bed with and they all had orgasms, including one woman who had never had an orgasm before. I think my skills are adequate and my dedication is serious and sincere. No one has complained, at least not until the second hour, when fatigue starts to set in. I'm not just going on their say-so about the orgasms, either. I suppose it's possible that a woman has faked an orgasm for me, but in most cases, some loss of control, increased flow of vaginal fluid, and the internal pulsations accompanying the orgasm are generally pretty convincing proof that they're for real.

And from a man with some good advice:

There's no consistent "right" way to go down on any one woman, let alone on all women you have the opportunity to go down on. Some women don't like a lot of pressure. Some don't feel it fully unless you press firmly. Start slow and respond to physical reaction and also to pleasure sounds and to direct verbal instructions. If a woman doesn't know what gets her off, you should be prepared to try lots of different approaches. If she does know and tells you, it's stupid not to follow direction, although being a little more experimental after the first orgasm should be okay."

Approach the pussy in your bed as if she still had secrets to tell you. She does. Rub your nose in her, lick her lips, and silently ask her, *What do you want?* She will let you know.

. . . .

DAY 99: FLIRTATION AND FOREPLAY MONDAY

New Lingerie Day

Who wears sexy new lingerie on Monday? A woman in a new relationship—or one who is cheating on her man.

Let him see you tenderly lift the new pieces out of their tissue. According to fashionistas, the thong is dead. Little boy shorts are the new trend—and the trend flatters all. Buy some lacy boy shorts and a matching bra.

Take your time wiggling into your new panties and bra.

If he doesn't ask, "Those new?"—say, "Like my new undies?"

Give yourself an extra spritz of perfume, including between the legs.

No, he will tell himself, *she couldn't possibly be having an affair—could she?*

....

 DAY 100: QUICKIE TUESDAY

The "Not in the Mood" Quickie

Sometimes he needs the pure sexual release, the dissipating of tension that only ejaculation gives a man. (And sometimes you need it more than he does.) This time, you are not in the mood or don't want to take the time for sex before going out, but don't say no to your man in need.

Whether you're dressing to go out or staying home, go into the bathroom alone, take a quick shower, and use a waterproof vibe to arouse yourself. Spray on fragrance and wrap up in a big towel or a silk robe.

Come up behind him and caress his cock (through his pants) into erection. Don't let him turn around until he is really hard.

Kiss him passionately as you guide him to the bed. Lay him down on the bed sideways across the mattress, his feet on the floor. Unzip his pants and straddle him.

Flex your PC muscles as you thrust, and pull the orgasm out of him.

....

👄 DAY 101: ORAL WEDNESDAY

Tea Bagging, His

In the days of royal harems guarded by eunuchs, when the master called a eunuch to help with his bath, he often expected a warmup called "nominal congress." The eunuch took first the master's balls and then his penis in his mouth. In slang terms, tea bagging is the art of sucking balls.

- Lick your way up his inner thighs while pulling down gently on his balls. Use your finger pads to "scratch" his thighs in the wake of your tongue.

- Now take his balls, one at a time, into your mouth. Roll them around and gently pull them down with your mouth.

(continued on next page)

- Hold his balls in your hand and run the tip of your tongue up and down the raphe, the line separating them. Strum the raphe. Now suck it.

- Return his balls to your mouth. Roll and pull while you work the shaft of his penis with your hand.

- You can bring him to orgasm through a combination of hand job and tea bagging—or give him a BJ.

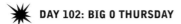

DAY 102: BIG O THURSDAY

The New Side-by-Side #1:
The Tight Embrace

The side-by-side positions are often "starter" positions. One partner is awake before the other. Awake—and horny. The best options for waking the sleeper are oral and side by side.

In the Tight Embrace position, adapted from the Kama Sutra position Transverse Lute, the couple lies in the traditional spooning position, with him facing her back.

Let's assume he is the aggressor (though it could as easily be her). He gently rolls her to her side and wraps his arms around her in a tight embrace. To give her better clitoral stimulation when he does penetrate her, he raises one leg and rests it on her thigh.

He enters her from behind and flexes his pelvic floor muscles. She will naturally pick it up and move in time with him. He doesn't begin thrusting until she is keeping his pace.

As they become more aroused, he loosens the embrace so they can prop themselves up on elbows. He pulls himself higher on her thigh and thrusts in this position until they are ready to move.

. . . .

 DAY 103: GET-YOUR-FREAK-ON FRIDAY

Playing the Dom

Years ago I hung out with some awesome professional dommes in researching a book called *Kink: The Hidden Sex Lives of Americans.* They know that many women secretly long to bring their man to his knees in submission to their sexual power. Here are their three secrets to successfully putting the role over:

1. Dress the Part

You don't have to buy an expensive leather or rubber catsuit, but you can't be a domme in your cozy sweats. Suggestions:

- A bustier or fancy bra

- Garter belt and black stockings, mesh or solid

- Sexy high heels

(continued on next page)

- Black lace panties

- Jewelry—large metal or animal print wrist cuffs, gold chains, even pearls can seem naughty in this context

- A flogger or whip in your hand (even if you don't use it)

2. Cop the Attitude

A domme is supremely self-confident and assertive. She is in charge. The submissive respects her because she *commands* respect, not demands it. Suggestions on how to project attitude:

- Stance—straight back, chest forward, legs slightly apart

- Voice—neither soft nor shrill, but firm, cadenced

- Mannerisms—hands behind back; restless flicking of the whip; pacing, which shows off your body in your hot outfit

- Eyes—cool, dispassionate, piercing

3. Give the Submissive What He (or She) Wants

The domme understands his fantasy and how to interpret it safely—and is careful not to spoil the scene for the sub by causing unwanted pain or humiliation. It's a game. Play it light.

....

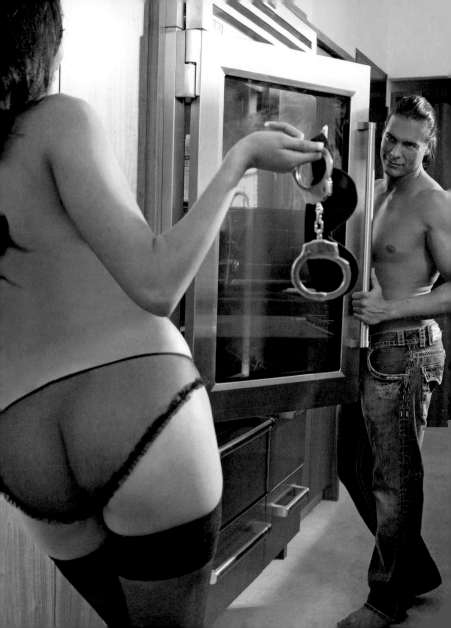

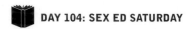 **DAY 104: SEX ED SATURDAY**

Chinese Sex #3: The Swinging Monkey

I love the name of this one! Don't you want to do it because it sounds like fun?

A variation on the Reverse Cowgirl, the Swinging Monkey is easy and elegant—and lends itself to ecstatic posturing.

1. He lies on his back with one leg raised, bent at the knee, foot on the bed.

2. She mounts him in the Reverse Cowgirl position, facing his feet—but she bends one leg and folds it over his bent leg so that her foot rests against his buttocks.

3. Now she puts her arms behind her and, bracing her weight on her hands, arches her back.

4. She thrusts by sliding back and forth on his penis.

A showy, beautiful position, the Swinging Monkey isn't good for the long haul. When you're both highly aroused, switch to a position that is easier to maintain and more conducive to orgasm.

....

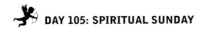 **DAY 105: SPIRITUAL SUNDAY**

The Ultimate Chakra Trick

You have probably heard about chakras, points of energy located in specific places in the body. Tantra teachers talk a great deal about chakras. I wrote a Tantra book that only refers to one chakra, which may be a record for the genre. This is a chakra trick you won't find anywhere else.

Chakra number five, located at the throat, is the chakra of creative expression. Some women can reach orgasm while performing fellatio without manual or oral clitoral stimulation. (Really, there is a physiological connection between the throat and the vagina.) If you are one of those women, this is your extra sexual energy zone. You feel the direct connection between your mouth/throat and genitals. There is a quick way to find out whether you have the potential to come while giving a blow job. Suck the head of his penis and pay attention to how your throat is responding. If it seems to quiver or vibrate faintly in time with your sucking, then you can do this.

As you are sucking him, breathe deeply and rhythmically. Imagine that your breath is a circle of fire inhaled into your nostrils, filling your mouth and throat, and exhaled through your genitals. Flex your PC muscle in time with your breathing and sucking.

It's a thrilling way to come, especially if your orgasm and his ejaculation happen simultaneously.

. . . .

The Fast Hot(ter) Shower

Not a quickie—but shower foreplay. Take a fast hot shower together.

If one partner is heading out of town for a few days, the hot shower is foreplay for the phone sex inevitably ahead.

Surprise your lover by getting into the shower with him, something you don't normally do unless you both have time to play.

Be all business—like sexual arousal is not on your mind at all. *Time-saving cleanliness* is the motive.

Turn your back to him and ask him to scrub. Then direct him to reach around and soap your breasts and pussy.

Rinse off. Turn him around and scrub his back. Reach around and soap his chest and his cock (erect by now).

Step out of the shower. Hurry off to get dressed. Wait for his dazed and glazed good-bye kiss.

....

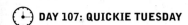

The Mutual Masturbation with Sex Toys Quickie

Add something extra to mutual masturbation: his and her toys.

His Toys

The vibrating cock ring is a silicone ring attached to a vibrating torpedo with battery pack. Give him a helping hand; slide it down his shaft.

Hand him a slender wand vibe and a finger vibe. Tell him you will hold that vibe against your cheek the next time you are fellating him. Or maybe you will use it on his balls while sucking his cock.

Now for the pièce de résistance: the Fleshlight. It looks likes a flashlight with cushy vagina lips on top. It feels as close to your pussy as he can get without going there.

Her Toys

Pull out your Rabbit vibe and rock it like this:

Flex your PC muscles as you gyrate your hips or squeeze your tummy muscles. Add a new twist by doing the scissors with your legs, crossing and uncrossing them as you flex and vibrate.

Switch to a finger vibe and give your clit extra stimulation and concentrated attention. Keep your eyes on his vibrations as you feel your own pulsing through your genitals. Can you really keep your hands off each other now? (It's okay to finish this quickie the old-fashioned way—with frenzied genital contact.)

....

The Rock 'n' Roll CJ, Hers

Perform cunnilingus, the CJ, to music, setting your pace to the beat. Plug in her favorite rock or hip-hop songs and get your groove on.

Put some cushions or a thick blanket down on the floor, smack in the middle of the bedroom or living room. She sits with her legs open as wide as is comfortable. He kneels in front of her—ready to bow his head in the position of worship to the rock princess. Or she can stand, her body swaying to the beat, with him sitting or kneeling in front of her.

Start with broad, lapping, up-and-down strokes of the entire vaginal area. Stiffen the tip of your tongue. Make a slightly stabbing move all around and up and down her clitoris (in time to the music, of course).

When the beat slows, use very light, very slow swirling moves around her clitoris, touching ever so gently on the head of it.

Now, add some light suction. Circle her clitoral shaft with your lips. Create the suction by inhaling through your mouth. The pressure on her clit will be gentle—and thrilling.

Add some equally gentle tongue action. You can increase the pressure of the suction and the speed of the tongue moves if she indicates she wants that. This move can produce earthquake-level orgasms in some women.

....

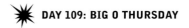 **DAY 109: BIG O THURSDAY**

The PC Factor

Kegel exercises to strengthen the PC muscle are the absolute bottom-line requirement for good sex. With a stronger PC muscle, you will have stronger, more intense orgasms. Women will have better control of his penis during intercourse and be able to do some amazing tricks by squeezing and relaxing her PC muscle around his penis.

If you aren't practicing Kegels, start *now*. Locate the PC muscle, part of the pelvic floor in men and women, by stopping and starting the flow of urine.

Begin with a Short Kegel Sequence

Contract the muscle twenty times at approximately one squeeze per second. Exhale gently as you tighten only the muscles around your genitals. Then release. Do two sets of twenty twice a day.

Then Add a Long Kegel Sequence

Hold the muscle contraction for a count of three. Relax between contractions. Again, do two sets of twenty twice a day.

Now Add the Push-out

After relaxing the contraction, push down and out gently, as if you were having a bowel movement with your PC muscle.

Create combinations of long and short sequences with push-outs. After a month of daily repetitions of 300, you should have a well-developed PC muscle. Keep it up by doing sets of 150 several times a week.

. . . .

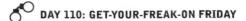 **DAY 110: GET-YOUR-FREAK-ON FRIDAY**

Playing the Submissive

In DS or BDSM games, the submissive is really in control. Nothing happens that she (or he) doesn't want. When dominant partners "push the limits" of their subs, watch carefully so that the experience doesn't turn into abuse.

Fueled by porn, the Internet, and powerful women looking for a good spanking, sex has become kinkier since I wrote *Kink: The Hidden Sex Lives of Americans* more than a decade ago. But don't play the submissive with strangers. Trust is the foundation of the game.

The dominant does the hard work. To play submissive for a night, first "surrender" control—putting your torment, and pleasure, in the hands of your partner, who is very clear on what you want. Some subs don a collar to signify they are ready to be dominated. Others say, "Do with me what you will, Master/Mistress." Settle on a signal or declaration.

Dress the part. For her, precariously high heels, a bra with the nipples cut out to facilitate the use of nipple clamps, and a waist-cinching garment to restrict her breathing somewhat and cause her genitals and breasts to swell. For him, a leather jockstrap or tight silk thong to show off his package. For both, leather or Velcro wrist and ankle bands, a blindfold, and a gag (optional).

Don't be afraid to use your safe word to halt or slow the game.

Realize the power of the submissive, and let it flash occasionally from your downcast eyes.

....

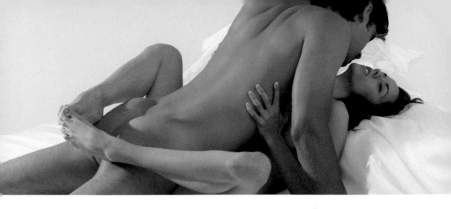

 DAY 111: SEX ED SATURDAY

French Lesson #1:
Pompoir (or the Butterfly Quiver)

The Butterfly Quiver was a specialty of priestesses and renowned courtesans in the ancient East. The French call it *pompoir*. The move is a variation on the PC flex. There are three Requirements:

1. Strong PC muscles

2. Slow thrusting

3. Good partner communication

When he is nearing ejaculation, she begins flexing her PC muscles in a continuous pattern of tightening and releasing, which replicates the pulsing of butterfly wings. It's most effective when he doesn't thrust too vigorously and leaves the movement largely to her. If she has a strong PC, he will feel like the ejaculate is being pulled from his body.

. . . .

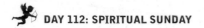 **DAY 112: SPIRITUAL SUNDAY**

New Intimate Position:
The Slow Spoon

The classic spoon position can accommodate more than one thrusting style. If he fits himself against her body, lifts and holds her buttocks, and enters her from behind, he can thrust energetically, especially if she is working with him. But spooning is also good for the slow ride—in this case, the really slow ride.

1. Lying on your left sides, place your right leg over the top of his and your left leg between his.

2. Now position yourself so your upper body is turned away from his, rather than spooned against it.

3. Put your right hand on the bed for leverage if that is comfortable for you. Or hold on to his right leg to control the thrusting.

This slight tweaking of the basic side-by-side position gives you extra clitoral stimulation. Once again, you will be pleasantly surprised at what a big difference a small change can make.

....

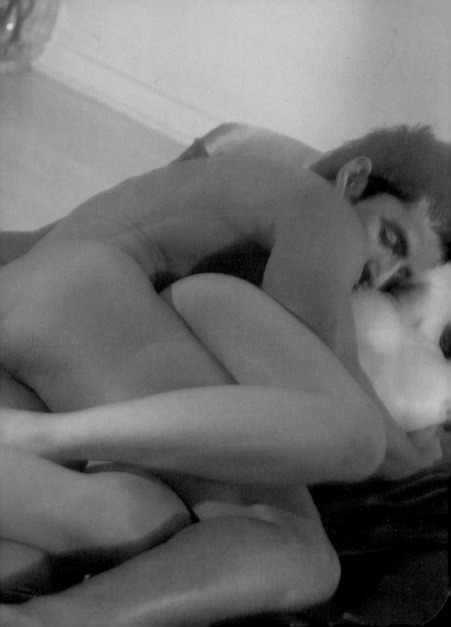

Erotic Poetry

Read—or write!—an erotic poem to your lover today.

Here's one for inspiration by one of my favorite poets, a Midwestern writer and teacher:

ORGASM

a stain spreads across the sheet

wet against the moment

movement against the grain

the wet deepens

the moment turns

electric into rhythm

rhythm into dark and free

there is no world outside this bed

there is no life but in my cunt

the moment turns

shatters

breaking truth into rhyme

there is no reason outside this time

this time

this torrent

this unrelenting wave

ROGWOLF

Reprinted with permission

....

The "Affair" Quickie

Pretend you are adulterous lovers who can rarely snatch more than fevered minutes together. A sudden opportunity for a quickie has just materialized. He's alone in his office for half an hour. She rushes across town to be with him. (Fortunately, she is not wearing panties.)

Embrace, kissing passionately, running your hands urgently up and down one another's body, hands in each other's hair as you grind your pelvises together.

Her need is as urgent as his—and she takes charge, pushing him down into his desk chair.

She straddles him, putting her thighs over the arms of the chair. The angle is fantastic for clitoral stimulation. She can hold on to the back of the chair or put her arms around his shoulders for leverage and support. His hands are free to ravish her body, especially her clitoris.

A variation: She sits on his lap, her back against his chest, using her legs for leverage. Again, he has both hands free to pleasure her.

....

The Rock 'n' Roll BJ, His

Go back to the middle of the room where he gave her the Rock 'n' Roll CJ last week (page 142). The music picks are his this time, and he will soon be too distracted to play air guitar or drums to the songs he loved in high school.

Let the spirit of his songs guide you as you put together a pattern of strokes. Get the beat going with two hands and a tongue move: Work his shaft up and down with one lubed hand. Caress his balls with the other, gently juggling them in their sac. Suck the head of his penis lightly while flicking your tongue across the frenulum. Run your tongue up and down the shaft. Now put both hands around his cock and work it to the beat. Suck the head. Suck the frenulum. Follow your hands on the shaft with your tongue. Keep it all moving as fast and furiously as the tunes play.

The secret to success in this BJ scenario is simple: Don't stop the tongue action 'til his song is sung.

....

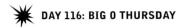

DAY 116: BIG O THURSDAY

The New Missionary #2:
Crossed Ankles

Occasionally, I hear from SexyPrime readers who say that a position did not work for them. Either they want to know what they did "wrong" or they want to persuade me that I am "wrong" and they are "right." It's sex, not mathematics. There are few absolutes when it comes to fitting two bodies together. This version of the missionary won't work for a woman with short legs or a tiny woman who is trying to wrap her legs around her BIG man.

When you wrap your legs around his waist, cross your ankles. That pulls him closer to you and deeper inside you. Very intense. If you wear a little sweetheart vibe—or insert the We Vibe between the two of you—you'll get all the clitoral stimulation you need, too.

If you are athletic, get into a shoulder-stand position. On his knees in front of you, he supports you by holding your legs up as he moves between them. Cross your ankles behind his neck. You have him in a gentle headlock. He has full access to your pussy and your clit with his cock and his hands.

. . . .

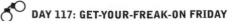

Body Painting

Almost everyone's inner child secretly loves to make a mess. Body paint-ing is a mess—but a nice sexy one. There are two ways to do it, one that will appeal to the neat-and-clean freak of the couple, the other to the more decadent lover. Isn't there usually one of each per couple? (And one who prefers morning sex and one who prefers night sex?)

Bathtub Paints

You can borrow them from the kids or buy your own adult version, but the product is the same. Only the packaging is different.

Paint one another in the bathroom. Hop in the shower and rinse it all off.

You may be so aroused by the painting that you linger a little longer in the shower or tub than is strictly necessary for the cleanup.

Flavored Paints

These come in chocolate and other flavors and are meant to be licked off, not washed off.

Put an old sheet on the bed. Turn your lover into a piece of edible art.

....

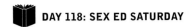 **DAY 118: SEX ED SATURDAY**

French Lesson #2:
The Parisian Gigolo's Kiss

When I was in Paris researching a book (*Sexational Secrets*), I met Michel, a gigolo. I was curious about his life—and more specifically, the sex. How good did he have to be to charge a Frenchwoman?

Michel insisted that his were likely no better than any good lover's sex moves. But his habit of paying intense attention, his playful charm, and his kiss! Being kissed by him was such a languid, erotic experience, I almost felt sated.

"A kiss is sacred," he said. "A man first enters a woman through her lips."

Here is the abbreviated version (in case you don't have two hours):

1. Kiss the inside of her wrist first. You will feel her pulse, which will heat up your lips.

2. Brush your lips across hers lightly. Pull back. Take her face in your hands. Put your lips on hers and press gently as you look into her eyes.

3. Explore her lips one at a time.

4. Close your eyes and kiss her passionately without inserting your tongue into her mouth.

5. French kiss her, using only the tip of your tongue to explore her tongue and dart in and out of her mouth.

. . . .

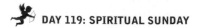

Expanded Orgasm, Lesson #1

An expanded orgasm extends beyond the genitals. You feel it in your groin, perhaps your buttocks or thighs. It lasts longer and stretches further than the average orgasm (not that there is anything wrong with the average orgasm).

First, practice lengthening and stretching your orgasm while masturbating, either alone or together.

His Stretching Exercise

Masturbate without ejaculating for as long as you can by stopping or changing strokes when ejaculation is imminent. Count the contractions you experience when you ejaculate—normally between three and eight. Next time you masturbate, try to delay ejaculation longer. With practice, you will increase the number of contractions you feel.

Her Spreading Exercise

Masturbate. As soon as you become highly aroused, use the other hand to massage with light, shallow strokes the area of the vulva, inner thighs, and groin. Imagine that you are spreading your orgasm throughout those areas. Continue the massage throughout your orgasm.

....

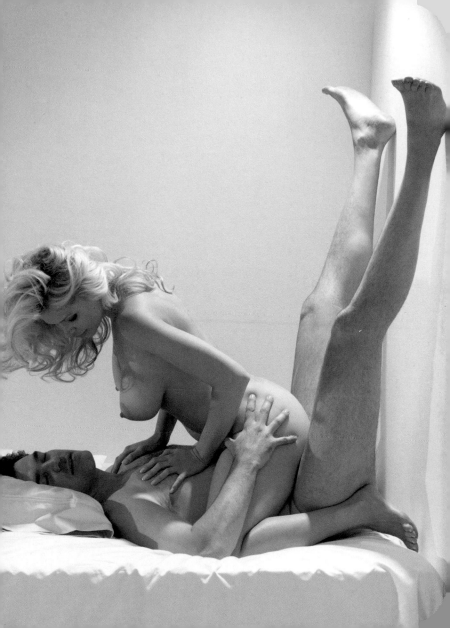

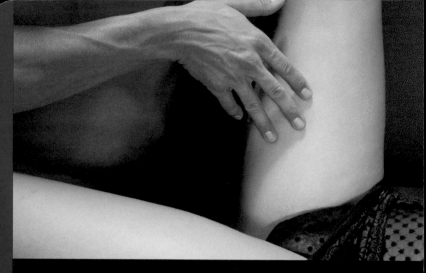

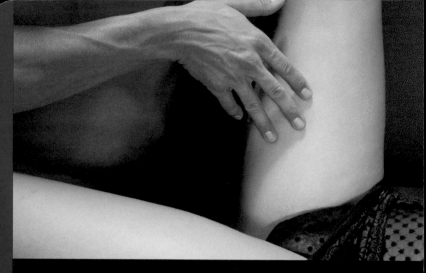 **DAY 120: FLIRTATION AND FOREPLAY MONDAY**

Spider Walk

An amusing light touch, Spider Walk is flirting with your finger pads. You can do this sitting at the table, standing, lying on the sofa, through clothes, or on bare skin. It stimulates the senses, without making the kids go "ew," like they do when they catch you in a kiss. The French call this game *Pattes D'Araignée*.

Walk your finger pads lightly over your partner's body and hair, the way a spider walks. Don't press down. You can also use the tips of your fingers if the nails aren't too long. Vary the pattern by, for example, walking up and down one arm, then up the next arm and around your partner's neck.

············

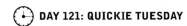 **DAY 121: QUICKIE TUESDAY**

Mental Foreplay

Dr. Gina Ogden introduced the concept of *starting on warm* in one of the best sex books ever written, *Women Who Love Sex*, about easily orgasmic women. It's the only way to get the most out of a quickie. The seduction takes place in your own head, and often the foreplay is in your own hands. You come to him ready.

Encourage Arousal Outside the Confines of Sex Acts

The tips and techniques in Flirtation and Foreplay Mondays are designed to encourage arousal, without any pressure to follow through. Often women shut themselves down unless they have "time for sex," meaning the thirty minutes to an hour that it takes for seduction, foreplay, and intercourse. Sexual is a state of being, not something you work up once or twice a week.

Focus on Your Sexual Fantasies

During the day on Quickie Tuesdays (and other days), fantasize sexy scenarios. Take a lesson from the guys. Don't censor your sexual thoughts. Enjoy them—and use them to build desire for your partner.

Indulge Yourself in Sensual Ways

Buy the good chocolate bar or a bunch of flowers. When you rub lotion into your hands or arms or body, appreciate how good your skin feels.

Stroke Your Clit

You don't need a reason to show it some personal love outside a masturbation session.

....

How to Suck #1:
The Long, Skinny Cock

You can perform all your best mouth moves with ease on a skinny cock. Anal intercourse is more comfortable. The one-hand hand job is effective. The length, however, can be challenging, especially if you don't want to deep throat. Here are some tips for getting the most out of what he's got.

Put More Hand in Your BJ

A good blow job is part hand job. Here are two ways for using your hands to trick his penis. Try Lou Paget's Ring and the Seal (page 102). Create a circle of thumb and first finger attached to your mouth so that it feels like he is going in deeper than he is. Dr Sonia Borg's A-OK solves the problem from the other end of the cock. Using the thumb and fore-finger of your left hand in the shape of an A-OK sign, glide them down to the base. Again, he feels like he is going deeper.

Flatten Your Tongue

Press it against the roof of your mouth, creating the sensation for him of hitting the back of your throat when he is not.

....

✳ DAY 123: BIG O THURSDAY

The Bend-Over Standing Position

The rear-entry standing position looks so hot in erotic photographs, but if the angle of penetration isn't right, it's lukewarm. Here's how to make standing sex feel as good as it looks:

1. With his legs comfortably apart, he stands behind her and holds on to her waist.

2. She leans forward so that her upper body is perpendicular to his; with arms outstretched to the sides, she holds on to a doorframe, braces against a wall, or leans into a dresser or another piece of furniture.

3. He squats slightly so she can lower herself onto him. If he is considerably taller than she is, she can stand on her toes, wear heels, or stand on a stool. The position allows her to influence the thrusting by pushing back against him, and the angle is good for G-spot stimulation.

4. A variation for the fit and supple: She bends all the way forward, touching her toes with her hands.

. . . .

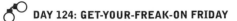 **DAY 124: GET-YOUR-FREAK-ON FRIDAY**

Porn Stars

Do you know that porn videos are honored at awards ceremonies just as mainstream films are? Actors and actresses, directors, and producers have their own version of the Oscars and the Golden Globes. Tonight, celebrate the best of erotic DVDs by acting out a scene (or more) from one of your favorite videos.

Really get into character and assume the personas of big stars, present and past, such as Ron Jeremy and the late Jamie Gillis, Jenna Jameson, Jamie Lynn, the Vivid Girls—or your favorite real people from amateur porn videos.

Some suggestions:

- The characters are easier to re-create than the scenes, because the pros do things on camera that the rest of us may not want to do.

- Women stars have big hair, obvious makeup, and fake nails, and wear very high heels.

- Men have the obvious equipment. (Put a sock in your jockstrap, if necessary.)

- Women moan and scream; men groan; everyone pants.

- You can simulate anal sex by talking dirty anal while doing vaginal rear entry.

- Women, when you catch the cum, put your tongue way out there.

....

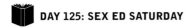 **DAY 125: SEX ED SATURDAY**

Advanced Arab Sex #1: Legs in the Air

Like many Eastern positions, this one is good for creating her arousal and sustaining intercourse, but it is not the best position for orgasm. However, it's easy to open those legs and shift positions when the moment is right.

1. She lies on her back and raises her legs (closed together) in the air.

2. He sits facing her, his legs open, one on either side of her body. He raises her legs further until they are vertical and rests them against one shoulder.

3. As he enters her, she closes her thighs around his penis, creating a tighter grip. (No penis fall-out here.)

The position does not allow for vigorous thrusting, but rather a slow buildup of erotic tension. She has both hands free to stimulate her clitoris and nipples.

....

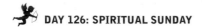 **DAY 126: SPIRITUAL SUNDAY**

The Letting-Go Exercise

What keeps you from fully enjoying your sexuality?

The number one culprit is negative sex attitudes, which can manifest in several ways. Women more than men are prone to judge harshly their own (and one another's) sexual behavior. But men have their own attitude traps, like the Madonna/Whore syndrome, which holds the wife/mother as too good for lust, while believing sexuality is all some other women have to offer.

Open a conversation with your man about the sexual attitudes that affect you and possibly him, too. Some of those negative attitudes include:

- Only young and beautiful women are sexually attractive.

- Intimacy is more important than sexual gratification for women.

- Men are always ready for sex and want more sex than women do.

- If you love each other, the sex will be rapturous, and if it isn't, you have fallen out of love.

Make this the day to get your hidden negative sex attitudes out on the table, where you can begin to let go of them. When you say them out loud, they sound ridiculous. But stuck in your head, they can do a lot of harm.

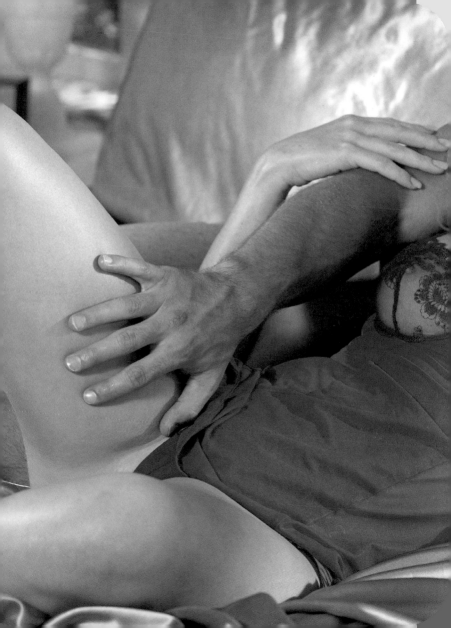

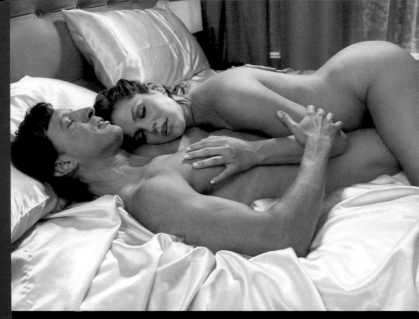

 DAY 127: FLIRTATION AND FOREPLAY MONDAY

Penis Push-Ups

You're already doing Kegels (see page 143) and your penis is growing stronger every day. Show off for her. Do a few penis push-ups while she is styling her hair or putting on her makeup.

Put a facecloth on your erection and move it up and down by flexing your PC muscle.

Build up to a damp facecloth and then a hand towel.

The Light-His-Fire Quickie

Booty Parlor—the purveyor of luxury sex product home parties—sells more than sex toys. The founder, Dana Myers, is the daughter of a Hollywood makeup artist who grew up watching her mother create not just beauty but also confidence in women. She aspires to do that with her own unique blend of sex toys and luscious lip glosses, bubble baths, and other treats. One of my favorite products is the Don't Stop Massage Candle. Use it to create a special quickie on this night when you want to please him alone.

Light the candle. Tell your man to lie back and enjoy the aphrodisiac fragrance while you kiss and caress him.

Once he has a hard erection, drizzle some of the warm oil from the candle onto his nipples. Use your thumbs in a circular motion to massage them.

Tweak and nibble his nipples as you drizzle warm oil at the base of his penis.

Lace your fingers together, holding his penis lightly inside them; use your thumbs (dipped in the oil) to massage in upward strokes on the sensitive underside of his penis from base to head.

Oil your fingers and give him a hand job, using a combination of his favorite strokes.

Let him come on your breasts. Mingle his cum with the oils from the candle and rub it into your nipples.

. . . .

How to Suck #2: The Short Fat Cock

Here is the cock you can deep throat—unless, of course, its girth is truly awesome. (That does happen now and then.) Some women consider this the perfect cock because it gives them the feeling of fullness where they want it during intercourse.

Suck Less, Lick More

Your mouth has to stretch wide to accommodate his width. That gets tiring fast. Alternate the sucking with licking, blowing, strumming, and swirling.

Nibble His Shaft

The Kama Sutra advised using teeth. Ouch. Try this instead: Cover your teeth with your lips and gently "bite" up and down the shaft. Finish by "biting" the head of his penis with those lip-covered teeth. He is meaty, after all.

Indulge His Desire for Showy Ejaculation

Finishing the blow job with your hands allows him to watch himself ejaculate—and gives you a break.

....

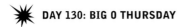 **DAY 130: BIG O THURSDAY**

The Clitoral Touch

In a survey on my blog, men reported more comfort with women giving themselves direct clitoral stimulation during intercourse than women did—with women under age thirty the most reluctant. These women want to know how they can come during intercourse without touching themselves, which is why I created the Orgasm Loop, a no-hands way of reaching orgasm that *works*. (You can also use a hand with it, if you like.)

Sadly, many women believe they have to sacrifice orgasm if there isn't a lot of time for foreplay, especially cunnilingus, before intercourse. You can come during intercourse alone, even during quickies. Some ways of doing that:

- Take charge of your own foreplay by using a vibe alone.

- Stop cunnilingus when you are on the edge of orgasm.

- Learn the Orgasm Loop, which speeds your orgasm in any situation (directions in *The Sex Bible, The Orgasm Bible, The Sex Bible for Women,* and *The Orgasm Loop*).

Another SexyPrime reader has a very useful tip for solving the problem: the guy should use his hand. He writes:

Put your hand down and around like you're going to pull her bottom up to you. Then snake that hand around, and you have full access to all of her. If her hand and your hand entwine in clit play, that's very hot.

....

Breast Intercourse

Most men do love breasts. Back in the not so ancient past before reliable birth control, savvy women sometimes satisfied their lovers between their breasts. It's quick and easy and gives you good sensations, too, if your breasts and nipples are highly sensitive. Plus, "breast fucking" feels a little freaky, always a good thing on Friday.

In either the woman-on-top or the man-on-top position, hold your breasts together around his erection, creating a snug, warm passage for his thrusting. As he is having intercourse with your breasts, tease the head of his penis with your mouth on the forward strokes. Quickly swirl your tongue around the head, flick the corona, or lightly suck the head. When he is ready to ejaculate, encourage him to give you a pearl necklace or shoot for your mouth.

....

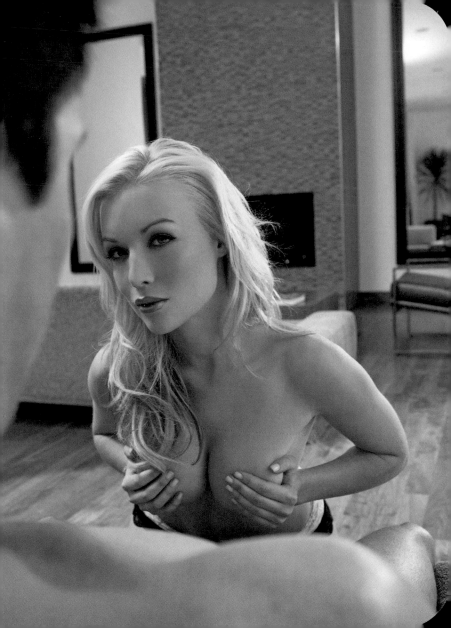

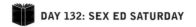

Advanced Arab Sex #2:
The Manner of the Bull

Sheik Nafzawi (see page 34), who created the original position thousands of years ago, said it was "the easiest of all intercourse methods"—with "easiest" being a relative term. I tamed this bull a little. While still retaining the character of the bull, it's a more user-friendly position now.

1. She lies on her front with pillows under her hips to raise her buttocks.

2. He approaches from behind, but not in the classic rear-entry position. Instead, he stretches his body along her back, fitting himself against her.

3. Once he has established the most comfortable and expeditious fit of their bodies, he inserts his penis into her vagina.

4. He holds on to her hip with one hand and wraps the other under her body so that he can stroke her clitoris as he thrusts.

5. The position limits his movement, sustaining his arousal and prolonging orgasm, while he brings her to one manually assisted orgasm after another.

....

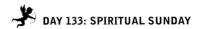 **DAY 133: SPIRITUAL SUNDAY**

Slow Sex: Extended Foreplay

Short segments of foreplay can last all day, keeping our bodies in a state of sustained arousal. At the end of the day, you will feel intensely connected to one another, exquisitely sensitive to every touch. The sound of your partner's breathing will reverberate in your genitals. And the sex will be explosive.

Some suggestions for foreplay time segments:

- Her breast and his nipple play

- Intense kissing

- Cunnilingus and fellatio—but not to orgasm

- Manual genital massage—again, not to orgasm

- Brief erotic massages

- Foot rubs and toe sucking

- Thigh play

- Anal play

....

Sexy Yoga, Pose #1

You can do this one, an adaptation of the Horse Gesture, together or alone. The anus and surrounding tissues are highly sensitive to erotic touch. But some people don't like being touched there. These exercises contract the anus to build heightened sensitivity throughout the area. You can get the feeling without the touching.

1. Sit in a cross-legged yoga position—or not, your choice. (It looks sexier if you do.)

2. Inhale deeply—and hold the inhaled breath.

3. As you exhale slowly, contract your sphincter muscles, pulling your anus up and in.

4. Repeat. Do a set of ten.

5. Now do a set of ten alternating the sphincter contraction with a PC flex.

············

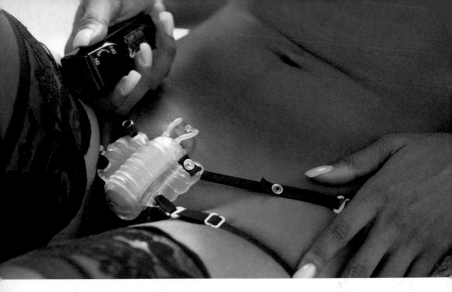

The Small Vibes Quickie

If she doesn't own a sweetheart vibe or a pair of vibrating panties, surprise her with the gift of your choice. Ask her to wear the vibe as foreplay, perhaps as you share a glass of wine or during dinner or while cleaning up the kitchen together.

When it's quickie time, take her in your arms, kiss, and fondle her. Vibrate her labia lips with a finger vibe as you do. Enter her from behind in a standing position and continue the finger vibe stimulation as you thrust. The double vibe action will bring her to orgasm quickly.

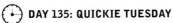

How to Suck #3: The BIG Dick

Unless you are in the porn industry, you aren't likely to encounter *many* BIG dicks—7 inches and more in length plus girth. But they are out there. You may have one in your own bed.

The disadvantages of a large penis are that anal sex is out for all but the most adventurous woman, intercourse positions have to be carefully calibrated, and gag reflexes are more easily triggered.

But the big one is beautiful, and you can learn to handle it.

Play with It Before You Take It Out of His Pants

It's so big you don't have to go looking for it. Massage his erection through his trousers. A tip from Dr. Sonia Borg: "Put your mouth around his clothed penis and make the humming sound coming from deep in your throat. This will send vibrations up and down his spine." Straddle him. Kiss him passionately. Open your shirt and free your breasts for his lips and hands. Press your vulva against his cock. Ride him so that you get good clitoral stimulation.

Suck Him in Smaller "Bites"

Starting at the head, work your way all around and down to the base in small sucking moves. Put your lips together as if you were going to kiss him, and pull in your cheeks slightly as you suck. Give special sucking time to the frenulum and the corona. Pay attention to his responses. Maybe you will find a secret place on his penis where no other woman has ever sucked so well.

Forget about Deep Throating

Don't worry about performing the ultimate deep throat. Take as much of him as you can into your mouth. Use the hand techniques for creating a "longer" mouth (page 158) and the "faux throat" tip (page 158). As long as your oral game is good and you are enthusiastic about his big toy, he will be happy.

. . . .

✸ DAY 137: BIG O THURSDAY

The New Missionary #3: Open Leg

I confess—this is one of my all-time favorite positions. Keep one side of the missionary position open, and you change the dynamics. Sometimes we want to be ravished; sometimes we want more control. In this variation, you have more control. It feels good and looks good.

Wrap one leg around his waist. The other leg is free so you can leverage the position, giving you greater impact on the depth and angle of penetration and the speed of thrusting.

Start with your leg bent, foot on the bed, and then move that leg into different positions as the mood changes. Some favorites: Throw it over his shoulder, lie partially on your side, or wrap it low beneath his buttocks. Use a small vibe or your hand or his hand to reach first orgasm quickly.

Make a dramatic pause just as he is about to come. If he's on top, grab his buttocks at the moment of orgasm, use your PC muscle to pull him in deeper, and then pinch or bite his nipple at the moment of his orgasm. Make eye contact with him as you're doing it.

. . . .

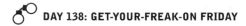 **DAY 138: GET-YOUR-FREAK-ON FRIDAY**

The Happy Hooker

Whether they have paid for sex or not, most men find the idea exciting—
even highly arousing. The Happy Hooker role-playing game may surprise
you. Try it. You might like it, too.

The Preparations

Negotiate the services and the fee in advance, over the phone. Blow job
only? Intercourse? Anal? Kinky? The rates rise according to the services
provided. He withdraws cash from an ATM.

She dresses the part of a high-class call girl—understated and elegantly
sexy clothing, pearls, classic high-heeled pumps, good lingerie. In her
classy little handbag, she carries condoms (which she will insist he wear)
and lube.

Turn the bedroom into a tastefully erotic hotel suite retreat with clean
sheets, flowers, champagne or wine on ice, and low lighting.

The Erotic Transaction

When she arrives at his room, he greets her, hands her the envelope of
cash, and pours her a drink. No kissing—unless they have negotiated
the Girlfriend Experience (costs extra for kissing and solicitous inquiries
about his day).

Showing off her assets, she undresses slowly. Depending on their
arrangement, she may or may not get naked.

She performs the agreed-upon services. Afterward they might share another glass of wine. When she leaves, she tells him to call the next time he is in town.

....

 DAY 139: SEX ED SATURDAY

The Desire Curve

Sexperts who promise you hot monogamy forever—or 24-hour orgasms—aren't being straight with you. Throw those books away. Understand the Desire Curve.

Created by therapist/coach and neuroscience researcher Nan Wise, the Desire Curve explains how and why our passionate desire for our lovers peaks and declines in eighteen months to three years. You have fallen off the high point of the curve, New Relationship Euphoria, because you have habituated to the lust drug cocktails created in your fevered brains.

From Nan, a few ways to trick the brain and make old sex feel new again:

- For God's sake, do *something* interesting/exciting/scary—both together and separately. Take a risk.

- Get kinky.

- Go back to college. Study a martial art. Do *something* to get your brains excited again.

- Switch your usual lovemaking steps and change the basic sex setup.

(continued on next page)

- Don't follow through to orgasm every time. "Sex" can be foreplay that gets you hot and bothered the next day, thinking about finishing it.

- "Give" your lover a sexual experience even if you aren't feeling much desire. This is a good time to perfect your erotic skills.

············

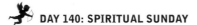 **DAY 140: SPIRITUAL SUNDAY**

Finding God through a Woman's Vagina

When I am looking for God, I look to the cock. Some men, artists and poets among them, find God through a woman's vagina. This is the essence of sacred sexuality. If, like me, you don't relate to most of the books and workshops on sacred sex, read a good book—and I mean, really, a *good* book. Many literary novels have erotic themes and graphic sexual content.

Some suggestions:

- *The Anatomist* by Federico Andahazi

- *100 Strokes of the Brush Before Bed* and *The Scent of Your Breath* by Melissa P.

- *The Lover* by Marguerite Duras

- *What I Have Written* by John A. Scott

- *Jeff in Venice, Death in Varanasi* by Geoff Dyer

- *Couples* by John Updike

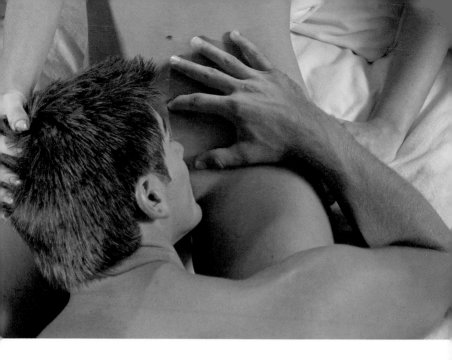

For inspiration:

When he opened his eyes, he saw that she was staring at his face and her lips were all tragic and her eyes were wet, and he was taken aback. It nearly made him stop. He should have looked at the eyes before now. What a waste! Looking into her eyes now, he felt drawn to something holy—a fire, life—it was sensational, he strove deeper inside her and felt a surge of excitement. "So you think you'll find God through a woman's vagina?"

—from *The Idea of Love* by Louise Dean

. . . .

Sexy Yoga, Pose #2

You can do this adaptation of the Root Lock alone or together.

1. Sit in the yoga position or lie on your back with knees bent. (If you do it together, face each other in the position or lie side by side.)

2. About halfway through a deep breath, contract your sphincter muscles.

3. Expand the breath and the contraction to the anus through the PC muscle supporting the pelvic floor and into the genitals. (Men will feel a pull in their testicles and women a quiver in the labia when they're doing this right.)

4. Do a set of ten.

5. Now do a set of ten, alternating this move with the PC flex.

....

The Phone Sex Quickie

Maybe you're both working late at your respective offices or one or both is out of town on business. Phone sex was conceived in just such erotically desperate times. But truthfully, phone sex in real life is often disappointing. Why? The partner initiating the call is in the mood and the other is distracted.

Make a date (with time limit) for a phone sex quickie. Here are some tips:

- Some people feel uncomfortable talking graphically. They may just need inspiration. Read or view sexually explicit material before the call. Consider it foreplay.

- The standard questions—What are you wearing? Are you touching yourself? Do you have an erection?—are good for creating visual images. You don't have to answer them honestly. ("Oh, I'm wearing my old gray sweatshirt and a pair of old panties"—TMI.)

- Talk each other through your last (or a favorite) hot quickie. Be specific. "Cup my ass and pull me onto your cock. Throw your head back and moan when I enter you."

- Put a lot of sexual energy and seductive emotion into your voice.

- Give yourself an electric boost. A small vibe, a vibrating cock ring—even porn playing silently on the computer screen—use whatever you need to intensify the experience.

....

How to Suck #4: The Standard Measure

Most men have an average-size penis, measuring 4 to 6 inches in length when erect with comfortable girth, neither hefty nor slender. You can do almost anything with the average penis. Doesn't that make it lovable?

Here are some suggestions for updating your BJ technique:

1. Be slow and deliberate with your tongue and lip moves so you can "hear" his penis telling you what feels especially good. Give that area extra attention.

2. Veer off the path of head, corona, frenulum, raphe—and see what happens. Some men have extra sensitivity in places you might be over-looking. The cock that had me dick-matized was exquisitely sensitive just below the corona and to the side of the frenulum (that little seam of skin on the underside of the shaft). I could make him come again sucking that place.

3. Pay attention to his balls. Gently pull them as you're sucking his cock.

4. Alternate lighter with stronger suction.

5. Use the underside of your tongue to lick up and down the shaft.

6. Put on your pearls! Let them fall down over his cock. Lightly twist them up and down the shaft of his penis while you're sucking the head.

7. Perform the BJ in a wildly exciting new scenario.

....

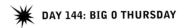 **DAY 144: BIG O THURSDAY**

The No-Fail Release-Him-Now Orgasm

He's tired; you're tired. He desperately wants sexual release. You are in a "none for me, thanks" place. True, he doesn't need your help to masturbate, but occasionally it's fun to lend a helping hand. Some women enjoy watching a man ejaculate. If you're naked while giving this hand job, let him come on your breasts. I worked this one out by watching porn films—and practicing—but the opening move is borrowed from Lou Paget.

1. Clasp your lubricated hands together, fingers interlaced, snugly around the shaft of his penis.

2. Move your hands up the shaft in one long twisting motion. Repeat the move back down the shaft.

3. Now vary that move by eliminating the twist.

4. When he has a firm erection, clasp your hands at the top of the shaft. Gently contract and release them around the shaft at approximately one second intervals. Keep doing this up and down the shaft, stopping at the corona, the rim where the shaft meets the head.

5. Alternate the twisting and contracting strokes until he is ready to ejaculate. Then hold him firmly in both hands, gently contracting them in time with his spasms.

6. Finish him off by running your thumb from the base of the shaft on the underside up to the head.

. . . .

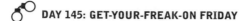

The Costume Box

Wherever you stash away your treasures, create a costume box and keep adding pieces to it. Clothing and accessories create an erotic mood. They project an aura that we step into—and become sexy characters.

Some suggestions:

- Vintage clothing store finds, such as old silk slips, patterned shawls, elbow-length gloves, Long strings of fake pearls

- Cheerleader skirts, kneesocks, pom-poms

- Letter jackets or sweaters

- Wigs and hats

- Garter belts and stockings, including patterned and mesh

- Leftover bits of Halloween costumes, such as a nurse's or maid's cap

- Feathered or sequined masks

- Old silk or velvet dressing gowns and robes

- Riding boots

- Props, from librarian glasses to cigarette holders—anything that sets a particular mood

- Old furs, including collars from discarded coats

....

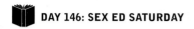

Indian Sex #1: The Kama Sutra Kiss

The Kama Sutra had little to say about oral sex, but it elevated kissing to an art form. There are nine types of kissing in the book. I have borrowed and adapted bits and pieces of the nine to create the ultimate Kama Sutra Kiss.

From "the initial kiss"—flirt with your lips, licking your lover's lips only with the tip of your tongue.

From "the tickling kiss"—run the tip of your tongue inside your lover's lips.

From "the rubbing kiss"—kiss softly, then rub your lips back and forth softly against his (hers).

From "passion feather kisses"—as your sense of urgency grows, give him (her) hot, fast kisses accompanied by moans, sighs, and gasps.

From "echo kisses"—one lover repeats the moves of another; for example, you suck her lower lip, she sucks yours.

From "licking kisses" and "biting kisses"—alternate the top and underside of your tongue when licking and add gentle bites of the lips.

From "the vibrating kiss"—in the midst of a passionate kiss, both lovers open and close their lips quickly and repeatedly, like two small fish.

From "the waterwheel kiss"—put your cheek to your lover's nose. Kiss his mouth. Insert the tip of your tongue and make a circular motion.

. . . .

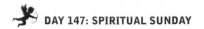

The Red Heels Kiss

Take him to your temple—your favorite shoe store—and build on yesterday's kiss. Let him help you pick out a new pair of red stilettos. In the shoe store, allow him to put them on your feet and caress your ankles as he does. When you get home, put on your stilettos and take charge of the kiss.

Hold his face in your hands and kiss him the way you want to be kissed.

Outline his lips with the tip of your tongue. Explore the tip and the edges of his tongue with the tip of your tongue.

If he tries to push his tongue into your mouth, gently but firmly push his face back. Circle the tip of his tongue with the tip of yours.

Repeat the above moves—and repeat again.

When you are aroused, thrust the tip of your tongue in and out of his mouth in a rhythmic, stabbing movement. If he's a fast learner, he will pick up the movement and give it right back to you.

Take one hand off his face and caress his neck. Let your hand run up and down his body as the kissing heats up.

Take his face in your hands again and run the tip of your tongue in circles just inside his lips. Tease those lips again and again with the circling tip of your tongue—the way you tease the head of his penis in the Silken Swirl (page 22). Suck his lips gently, one at a time.

Now melt into his arms and let him do you. Red Heels Sex . . .

....

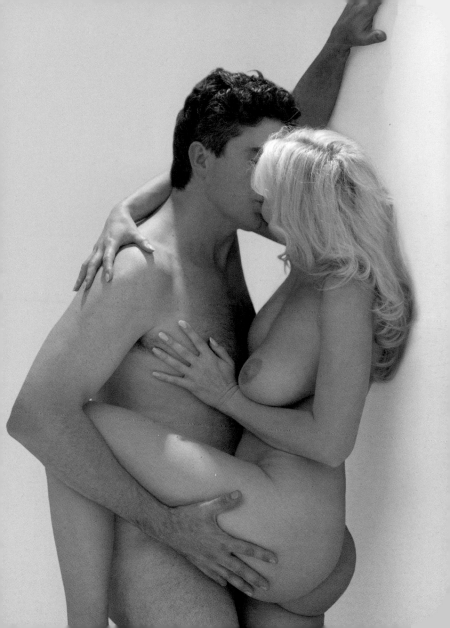

Sexy Weight Moves #1

Women, buy a set of 5- or 7-pound hand weights, men a set of 10- or 15-pounders. Keep them in the bedroom, tucked under the bed or inside the closet. Put together a simple routine of strength and toning moves. Many of them feel sexy and look just as good. Do them in your underwear or nude. Yours won't be the only blood circulating faster.

The Squat/Bicep Curl is a good one to put suggestive thoughts in your lover's mind.

1. Stand with your legs comfortably apart. With arms close to your body, hold a weight in each hand.

2. As you curl the weights up, squat. Weights back down, straighten legs.

3. Do a set of at least 20 and build from there.

The New Kitchen Counter Quickie

In the classic Kitchen Counter Quickie, she sits at the edge of the counter and he stands in front of her. It's a great position for a little woman with a big tall lover. (I speak from personal experience.) This variation also opens up possibilities for shorter men and taller women.

He sits, naked from the waist down, at the edge of the kitchen counter.

She stands on a sturdy box or stool so her pussy is even with his cock.

He supports her by holding her in his arms, one or both hands clasping her buttocks, as she wraps one leg loosely around his waist and mounts him.

If the kitchen counter is wide enough to accommodate the couple in a sitting position, she can wrap both legs around his waist and sit down on his erection.

....

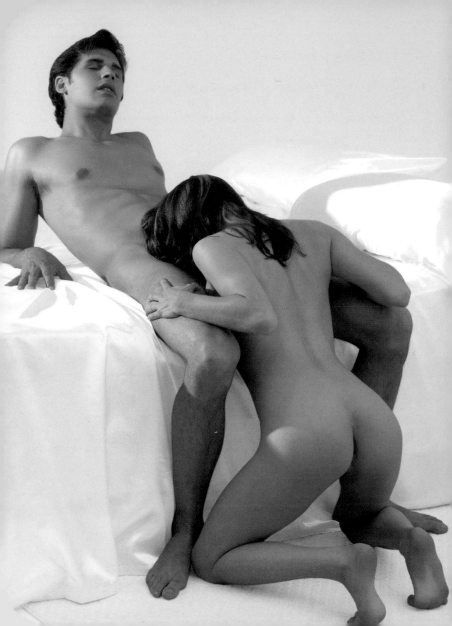

How to Suck #5: The Semierect Cock

Your mouth alone cannot raise the limp. Combine mouth moves and firm hand action.

Hold his penis firmly in one hand. Take it into your mouth, moving the top third of the shaft in and out. Use the fingers of your other hand to stroke his perineum in a light, tickling, come-hither fashion

When he is at least semierect, use both hands to do a circular twisting motion; at the same time, swirl your tongue around the corona.

Strum the frenulum. Alternate the swirl with flicking your tongue back and forth across the corona.

Continue the hand move while taking his testicles into your mouth, one at a time, and sucking lightly. Flick your tongue lightly across his perineum. Go back to his penis and alternate swirling, flicking, and sucking.

Don't take his penis too far into your mouth or you won't be able to pull off the suction. And don't make it look like work. If it begins to feel like work, stop and tell him you are so aroused from sucking him that you need some oral attention, too. Some men tell me that nothing gets them erect faster than performing cunnilingus.

. . . .

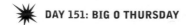 **DAY 151: BIG O THURSDAY**

The Masturbation Show

Sometimes he is just not in the mood—to do it, that is. He's always in the mood to watch.

Put on a very sexy shirt or lacy tank top and nothing else, except perhaps black lace-topped thigh-high stockings and heels. Assume a provocative position with your back against the headboard, legs bent and open at the knees, ass elevated by a pillow or two. Give him a view.

Place two fingers in an inverted V straddling your clitoris. That hand position is good for encouraging your orgasm and also for showing him what you've got.

Throw yourself into masturbation with abandon. If you have the kind of headboard that permits it, put your hand over your head and grasp a rung or bedpost. Thrust your pelvis forward. Pant and moan.

Add some flashy moves, such as:

- The Figure Eight: Use one finger to glide up, over, and around your clitoris as if you were tracing the number eight.

- The Two-Finger Thrill: Hold two fingers parallel on either side of your clitoris. Run them up and down and then sideways.

- Vibe Play: Use one of the contour vibes or a small bullet vibe or the Pocket Rocket—any vibe that will give you a good clitoral buzz without blocking his view of your pussy entirely.

....

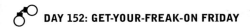 **DAY 152: GET-YOUR-FREAK-ON FRIDAY**

The Naughty (Male) Nurse

The woman plays the nurse (and the man the doctor) in the classic role-playing fantasy. Give it a new twist. He is the nurse; she is the wealthy, demanding patient.

The Preparations

Borrow or buy a set of scrubs or wear lightweight sweat or martial arts pants with a matching shirt. Create an ID badge on your computer.

Put crisp white sheets on the bed. Don't forget the hospital corners. Fill small glass bottles with M&Ms, jelly beans, or other candies to look like "medicine." Buy a children's doctor or nurse play kit.

The patient eschews the hospital gown in favor of a short nightie. Very short. She has a bell for summoning the nurse—and uses it often.

Agree on her medical complaint, perhaps she needs some physical therapy?

The Game

He performs a routine checkup of her vital signs, which necessitates taking her pulse, examining her tongue, and checking her reflexes—providing opportunities for her to stretch out her arms and legs in interesting ways.

She repeatedly summons him with the bell seconds after he leaves her bedside. She may need her back scratched or a leg cramp massaged. And she has so many questions and concerns: Do my breasts feel normal, Nurse? Is there a rash on my ass? My pussy feels cold.

(continued on next page)

In gratitude, she kisses him. In deeper gratitude, she caresses the erection she sees inside his pants.

"I can't sleep unless I have an orgasm," she tells him.

....

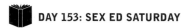 **DAY 153: SEX ED SATURDAY**

Indian Sex #2: Scratches and Bites

The *Ananga Ranga*, one of the great Indian love manuals, like its inspiration the Kama Sutra, devotes quite a bit of attention to the arts of scratching and biting. A little of that erotic violence judiciously applied in the throes of passion can take your arousal higher. Is sex sometimes "boring" or "routine"? Be an animal.

Some techniques adapted from the Indian love manuals:

The Upper Lip Nibble
In this gentler, kinder version of *uttaroshtha*, take his lower lip between your teeth without biting down. Hold it there for a few seconds. Now do the same with his upper lip. Finally, graze your teeth very lightly across his upper lip.

The Hard Kiss
Modeled on the Coral Kiss, this kiss only hints at the power of teeth on flesh. He lets her feel his teeth while he is sucking her lips one at a time, and then again briefly as he kisses her passionately with her mouth closed.

The Cupped Scratch

Make sure your nails are filed smooth. Cup your hand and use your nails very lightly in a tickling scratch on breasts, belly, back, buttocks, and inner thighs. If your lover wants a little more vigorous tickling scratch, that's good, but wait to be asked for "more" before you give it.

. . . .

 DAY 154: SPIRITUAL SUNDAY

Hearts Breathing

Synchronized breathing—together with eye gazing—intensifies any sexual encounter. Try breathing so that your hearts seem to be in time. Initially, you will feel awkward. Resist the temptation to make a joke. Give it ten minutes and you will be a convert.

1. Sit on the bed with your legs crossed, facing each other.

2. He puts his right hand over her heart. She puts her right hand over his heart. Her left hand covers his right; his left hand covers her right.

3. Breathe in unison while gazing into each other's eyes.

4. Gaze, breathe; gaze, breathe. Don't talk. After a few minutes or five, you will look at your partner's face and see a change. Facial muscles relax. The whole face seems to open up to the lover.

5. As you breathe and gaze, imagine love flowing from eyes to hands to hearts. You will be surprised by the intensity of the connection you feel to one another now.

. . . .

Sexy Weight Moves #2

Pull out those weights again—and turn yourself (and your lover) on. If you have a full-length mirror, stand in front of it as you do this one.

The Row-It-All-the-Way-Up

1. Stand with your legs comfortably apart, hands at your sides, a weight in each hand.

2. Bring your hands together with the weights touching in front of your body.

3. Bend from the waist. The weights remain touching as you lower them to the floor.

4. In a rowing motion, pull them back up to your waist.

5. Turn your arms so that your hands are facing in and raise the weights over your head.

6. Come back to your waist and position the weights together again.

7. Do a set of at least 20 reps.

....

The "Favorite Friend" Quickie

We all have a "favorite friend" fantasy—the one that gets your game on fast. The fantasy may be of another lover, a "taboo" sex act, a "zipless fuck" with a stranger, or any sex fantasy. We revert to it in masturbation when we want to come in a hurry. Sometimes we daydream it when we're tired or lonely. Few people admit it, but almost everyone has brought the fantasy into his or her lover's bed.

You can love your partner and generally have good, even great, sex with him or her and still sometimes need to fantasize. That's life. And this is one of those days.

Don't waste time feeling guilty about it. Unless you habitually use this fantasy, to the point where you can't come without it, there is no problem. But don't share it with your partner. Why? One, a fantasy often loses the power to arouse us when we share it. Two, though she or he also likely has a fallback fantasy, she or he may not like it that you do.

Incorporate some elements of the fantasy encounter into your quickie. For example:

- Does your favorite friend involve a little bondage and discipline? Ask your lover to slap your ass—hard.

- Is it set on a beach or desert island? Turn up the heat or turn off the AC.

- Stranger encounter? Keep your eyes closed.

. . . .

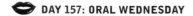

The CJ with Hands

Put your hands into this CJ—but don't go for the obvious place, the G-spot. Instead of lying between her outstretched legs, sit at her hip. Stroke her vulva.

Gently open her legs and run your hands in broad strokes up and down her inner thighs. Scratch lightly with your fingernails. Run your finger pads in a Spider Walk (page 156).

Get up on your knees and bend over her vulva from the sideways position. Part her labia and lick her lips slowly as you continue to stroke her thighs and outer lips.

Use your face. Nuzzle and rub her clitoris and surrounding tissue with your nose and cheeks as you stroke her labia.

Combine each oral move with a hand move that echoes it. For example, pretend your tongue is a flickering flame lapping at the shaft of her clitoris and occasionally flicking the head as your fingers flutter back and forth between her labia.

Put the tip of your tongue against the shaft of her clitoris. Move your head slightly back and forth while you move your fingers back and forth in her labia.

Lick the tissue on one side of her clit and stroke the other with your finger.

When she is close to orgasm, give her the clitoral touches that work best for her. And now you can go for the G-spot.

....

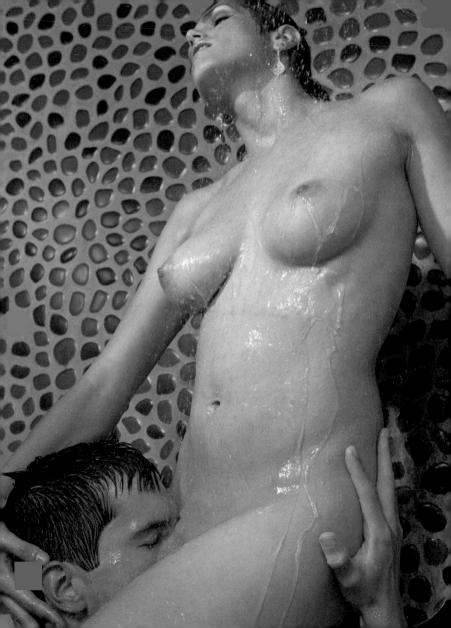

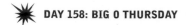 **DAY 158: BIG O THURSDAY**

The Pressure Orgasm

There is a type of female orgasm rarely discussed. Dr. Betty Dodson, the "Mother of Masturbation," defines it as a pressure orgasm, resulting from indirect stimulation or "pressure" to the clitoris and surrounding area. To experience a pressure orgasm during masturbation, try one of these:

- Squeeze your legs together as you contract your PC muscle.

- Rub back and forth against something hard, such as a padded head-board or chair arm.

- Straddle a folded bath towel and work that back and forth between your legs (a popular form of masturbation, especially in college dorms).

Can you come this way? If so, you can translate that skill into inter-course. Position yourself so that you are grinding into your partner as he thrusts.

....

 DAY 159: GET-YOUR-FREAK-ON FRIDAY

His Striptease

A former Chippendales' dancer says the secret to stripping for women is eye contact. "It is the reverse for women strippers who make minimal eye contact with the male audience, even when they're giving them lap dances," he says. "Women want to look into your eyes and see desire and fantasize that it is for them."

The Preparations

Practice taking off your clothes to music. Stepping gracefully out of slacks is an art. Don't even think about trying it with tight jeans.

To prolong the tease, wear a tie and cufflinks, if you have them.

Add an unexpected element by wearing a pair of her silk panties under your slacks or a satin male G-string.

Set the mood you want to create with lighting, music, and accessories. A bowl of roses on the table delivers a different message from a bowl of peanuts.

The Striptease

Make it last a little longer by removing items from your pockets. Toss your wallet and keys onto the bed in a suggestive way.

When you take your belt off, whip it around in the air.

Leave your shirt unbuttoned and open while you remove your slacks.

Give her the opportunity to touch your bare chest before you finish stripping.

And don't forget: Seduce her with your eyes and your body.

....

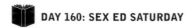

Indian Sex #3: The Wide-Leg Position

The missionary, or man-on-top, position may be the most favored in Western society—as it was in ancient Arabia—but the Indian love experts held them all in high esteem. There are more variations for the missionary in the Kama Sutra than for other positions because the author wisely realized that women needed adaptations to the basic pose to provide them opportunity for orgasm. I hope you will read more about the Kama Sutra and also read Sir Richard Burton's translation of it; enlightenment comes in many forms and has occurred along the historical continuum.

1. Lying on her back, she leans her head back, arches her back, and opens her legs wide. She can bend one or both legs for support and leverage. The position thrusts her pelvis forward.

2. He kneels between her legs. After he enters her, he flattens himself against her upper body without putting weight on her. His weight is supported by his knees and one arm.

3. He reaches around with the other hand and stimulates her clitoris as he thrusts inside her.

....

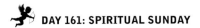 **DAY 161: SPIRITUAL SUNDAY**

The Spiritual BJ

My pal Steve Otero emailed me a post from Sensuous Sadie's blog: "The Spiritual Blow Job (No, Really!)." Her dominant taught the submissive Sadie how to perform a longer BJ as an act of worship. Although I am no submissive, as a devotee of the cock, I found this an appealing idea. I have a special relationship with the penis—or the magnificent ones capable of dick-matizing me—that is unsullied by whatever relationship I do or don't have with its life support system, the man.

Here are some of Sadie's tips for prolonging a BJ:

- Make prolonged eye contact and synchronize your deep breathing. Matching your breathing to his automatically slows him down, at least for a bit. And it intensifies the feeling of intimacy by making you feel more connected to one another through the mutually shared miracle of his dick.

- Suck less; lick more. The sucking brings him to orgasm.

- Use the Squeeze technique. Lightly squeeze the head of his penis when he is near ejaculation to hold him back. But don't do that more than two or three times a session.

- Oil your breasts. Lie back and put his penis between them. Squeeze your breasts together. As he thrusts, lick or lightly suck the head of his penis on the forward stroke.

....

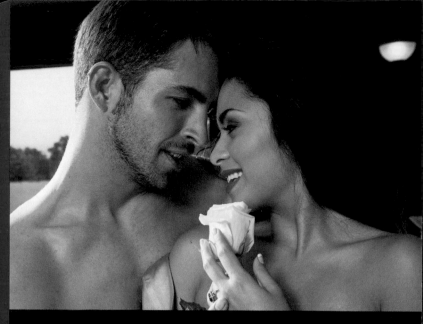

DAY 162: FLIRTATION AND FOREPLAY MONDAY

The Heart Touch

Placing a hand over your lover's heart is an incredibly effective move for such a small investment of thought and energy.

Take an extra few seconds after the hurried good-bye kiss and put your hand over his beating heart. Hold it there as you look into his eyes. With this quick gesture, you are reestablishing the intense intimate connection of Hearts Breathing (page 175).

If somebody doesn't say "I love you" I would be surprised.

....

The Voyeur Quickie

This story comes from a SexyPrime reader.

Before my husband and I were married, we lived together in a Manhattan apartment on the edge of the Gramercy Park area. We could look right into the windows of apartments across the street—or they into ours—which is how things are in the city. Occasionally, we caught glimpses of people undressing or groping for one another before heading off presumably to the bedroom. I've heard about overweight middle-aged couples having sex in swings with the drapes open, but it's probably an urban myth.

One night we were cuddled up on the sofa watching TV. I glanced out the window and saw a tall woman with a smokin' body standing naked except for a glittery necklace, legs apart, right up in front of her window—masturbating!

I poked my boyfriend. He looked up and had an almost instant erection. As we watched, she spread her legs wider, licked her lips, wet her fingers in her mouth. She circled her clit with her fingers in exaggerated motions, played with her nipples, and finally threw her head back as if she were in the throes of orgasm.

I unzipped my guy's pants, pulled out his cock, and we had the hottest quickie of our lives.

If there are no opportunities for watching the neighbors masturbate from your house, then watch some porn together.

. . . .

The Perineum Orgasm, His

The perineum (the space between his anus and the base of his testicles) is incredibly sensitive in some men, but not in others. If you haven't explored this area together, do so now.

Stroke his perineum during oral or manual foreplay. If he is responsive, go back there when he is highly aroused. As you are sucking his cock or giving him a hand job, keep one hand free to play with the perineum. Stroke it. Press your thumb or finger pad lightly into it.

When he is on the brink of ejaculation, hold his thighs apart and lower your mouth to his perineum. Flick your tongue rapidly back and forth across that area. Now press your thumb lightly against his perineum—gauging the pressure by his response—as you continue flicking your tongue. This drives some men wild, but affects others not at all.

. . . .

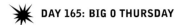

DAY 165: BIG O THURSDAY

Her Multiple Os #2: Sequential

Women can experience four types of multiple orgasms. On page 71, I explained compounded single orgasms, perhaps the most common. They are separated by sufficient time for arousal to have subsided substantially between orgasms.

Sequential multiples are orgasms that are fairly close together—any-where from two to ten minutes apart—with little interruption in sexual stimulation or level of arousal.

Women most often report them during cunnilingus. Her lover can encourage them by:

- Constant, concerted stimulation on and around the clitoris (which does not work for every woman)

- Alternating sucking the clitoral area with licking and flicking the shaft

- The Flame: Pretend the tip of your tongue is a candle flame. In your mind's eye, see that flame flicking in the wind. Move your tongue rapidly around the sides of her clitoris, above and below it, as the candle flame moves.

....

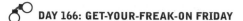

Edge Play

In DS or BDSM terms, "edge play" can refer to the dominant taking the submissive to the edge of his or her limits. But that is not how I am using the term here.

Sex researchers Dr. William Masters and Dr. Virginia Johnson concluded decades ago from their research that the outer third is the most sensitive part of the vagina—as the first third is the most sensitive part of his penis. That is likely true for most people. Yet men and women both crave deep penetration.

Use the head of his penis as her foreplay. Then have intercourse with only the first third of his penis. Keeping him at the edge will make both of you ravenous for deeper penetration, and it will feel so good when you let yourselves go there.

- Take the head of his penis in your hand and rub it against your clitoris. Use it in creative ways, like pressing the side of the head against the shaft of your clit.

- Don't let him penetrate your vagina until he is begging for that.

- He takes shallow thrusts.

- She periodically removes his penis from her vagina and uses it to stroke her clitoris again.

....

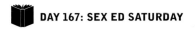 **DAY 167: SEX ED SATURDAY**

Japanese Sex #1: Silk and Sake

The ancient Japanese were very passionate about seizing their sexual pleasure. Like other Eastern practitioners of the erotic arts, they believed that great sex was a high value that required good sexual technique, combined with imagination and something you might not expect, a sense of humor. Indulge in a night of silk and sake—your introduction to sex in the ancient Japanese way.

The Preparations

Wear flowing and luxurious garments meant to be kept on during sex play.

Buy a calligraphy pen from an art store, aromatic oils, a single orchid spray, and sake, potent Japanese wine, and serve it warm.

Each partner researches ancient Japanese sexuality and comes prepared with either five facts or an erotic poem or story.

Focus on Foreplay

Take the calligraphy pen (or a firm feather), dip it in oil, and lightly touch some of your partner's pleasure points, including nipples, breasts, groin, the midpoint of the perineum, and the Cinnabar Field, seven points from the navel to the pubic symphysis, at the front of the pubic bone above the genitals. Imagine a line connecting the navel and the pubic symphysis, with five additional points spaced more or less equidistant from the others. Using hot, feathery kisses, begin at your lover's mouth, trail down her (his) neck, and kiss the pleasure points.

. . . .

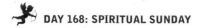 **DAY 168: SPIRITUAL SUNDAY**

Kundalini #3: Energies Rising Together

On page 83 you awakened your kundalini energies, and on page 107 you connected them in sexual intercourse. Try raising those energies through your genitals and up into your bodies and heads. It will feel like very intense intercourse with a spiritual climax.

There is a scientific explanation behind this. Any form of deep breathing increases oxygen levels and forces more blood into your genitals. That, in turn, encourages your brain to create a stronger lust hormone cocktail.

Begin fire breathing with foreplay. Imagine you are moving the heat into and out of each other's bodies, not just your own.

Keep up the fire breathing during intercourse. Don't worry if you lose a cycle or two. Just pick it up again, especially at the point of orgasm.

Continue stroking, fondling, even stimulating one another's genitals after orgasm.

Lying in one another's arms, make upward strokes with your palms along your lover's spine. Imagine you are raising the sexual energies into your hearts and finally your heads.

....

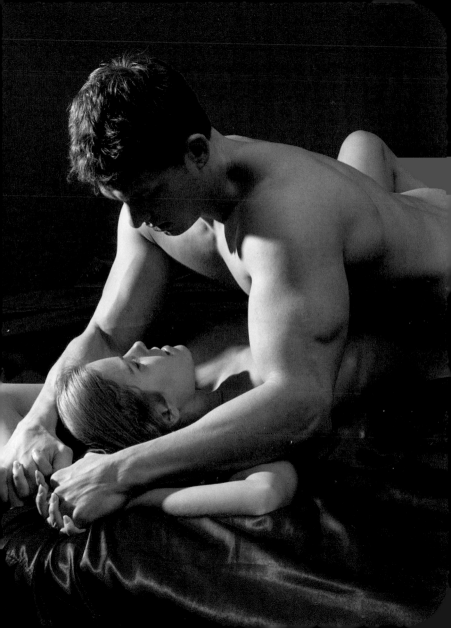

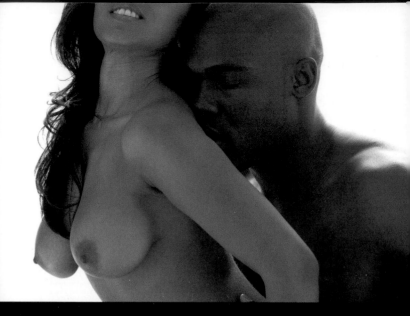

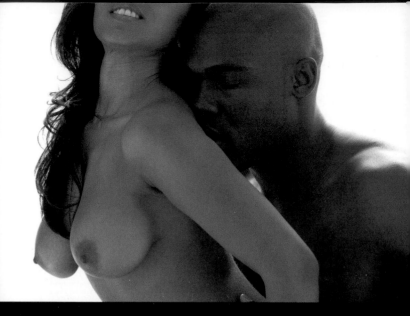 **DAY 169: FLIRTATION AND FOREPLAY MONDAY**

Sharing Grapes

Keep a bag of grapes in the freezer. Frozen grapes are satisfying on so many levels, including as a low-calorie natural substitute for sorbet. The next time you're cooking together, put a small bowl of them on the counter between you.

Take turns popping the grapes into one another's mouths.

Take time for quick kisses—and transfer a frozen grape in the kiss.

Whisper some naughty suggestions about what else you might do with a frozen grape—or your cold mouths.

....

"Up Against the Wall" Quickie

Get out the fur-lined handcuffs and water pistols. Today you play cop and apprehended suspect (the grown-up version of "cops and robbers"). If you can find a holster for your gun and lube, wear it slung low over bikini panties (his or hers).

The Setup

The cop is waiting in the dark behind the bedroom door. Her sweetheart vibe is doing its job on her clitoris. Gun drawn, handcuffs attached to her holster, stilettos ready for action, she calls out, "You're under arrest" when the suspect opens the door.

If the room is pitch dark—no moonlight, no light streaming in from the bathroom—she turns on a small lamp so the perp can admire her uniform of heels, holster, and panties.

Brandishing her pistol, she says, "Up against the wall, hands up high!"

The Quickie

Pat him down. Put your hands on his concealed weapon, the bulge in his pants. Tell him you have to inspect it. Unzip his pants. As he is standing with his pants around his ankles, work his cock up and down with one hand.

You can cuff his hands behind his back, sink to your knees, and disarm that no-longer concealed weapon with a blow job, or he can knock the gun out of your hand, kick off his pants, order you to get down on all fours, and take you from behind.

....

"69" with Alternating Tongues

I often use that one-line zinger: "The last time anyone had a great time doing '69' was in '69." Amusing, isn't it? Truthfully, the mutual oral sex position usually looks better (onscreen) than it feels. Both the giving and the receiving of oral pleasure are intense pursuits.

If you are intensely involved in receiving, how can you be getting your best oral game on? Try taking turns. Here's how:

Agree to the basic rule: When one is licking and sucking, the other's mouth is in repose.

Use your signature oral moves, the ones that work best on your lover, and save new lick tricks for another time.

Start slow, with the:

- Lollipop Lick for him: Begin by licking up the raphe (the line between his testicles), up the center of the shaft, and finish with a swirl of the head.

- Ice Cream Cone for her: With a flat, wide tongue, lap her labia lips and up to her clitoris.

Take turns bringing one another to high arousal, then backing off.

Keep alternating tongues until one partner begs for release.

....

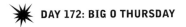 **DAY 172: BIG O THURSDAY**

The "Go-for-Long" O Tricks

A frequent question from male SexyPrime readers is: "How can I last longer in intercourse both for myself and my partner?" Both men and women are disappointed when he comes "too fast." They want to give her a chance to reach orgasm during intercourse, too. Here are the three best technique tricks:

1. Flex your PC muscle. (Practice your Kegel exercises. Strengthening the PC gives you more control over your ejaculatory process so you can sustain thrusting longer.)

2. Slow your breathing. Take slow deep breaths as you are thrusting. Your body will slow the thrusting in time with your breathing.

3. Hold your penis at the base as you're thrusting. After a few strokes, pull out, slide your hand up and lightly squeeze the head, thrust a few more strokes again, repeat. Most men use the Squeeze (the classic Masters and Johnson technique) when they feel ejaculation is imminent. Don't wait that long. Three or four light squeezes should help you sustain intercourse.

Some people believe "the science of sex" is cold, and that passion, like love, conquers all. It doesn't overcome bad technique. Erotic skills facilitate the flow of passion from one lover to another. Being good in bed may not guarantee you will find true passion, but you will have pleasurable sex, with nobody going to sleep or home unsatisfied.

....

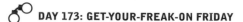 **DAY 173: GET-YOUR-FREAK-ON FRIDAY**

Female Ejaculation

Some women are "squirters," at least occasionally, most likely with G-spot stimulation. Many Western sex experts dismiss the "ejaculate" as merely a gush of fluid composed of urine and copious vaginal secretions. Others believe it is fluid from the Skene's glands, a string of several masses of tissue, embedded in the urethra, which, when stimulated sexually in some women, release the fluid into the urethral canal.

Men ejaculate sperm from the testicles via tubes that go through the prostate gland, where the sperm mixes with seminal fluid, a very clear process that everyone understands. There is no question that whatever this fluid is, it is not the female equivalent of seminal fluid. Strictly speaking, there is no female ejaculate or ejaculation.

Devotees of Amrita, who believe that female ejaculation is sacred, consider the fluid to be the "nectar of the goddess." If not ejaculate, then what is it? I lean toward the Skene's glands theory because it makes the most sense to me.

Female ejaculation isn't exactly a technique. If you want to try to make it happen, follow these tips:

- Drink a lot of water in preparation, but don't have sex with a full bladder.

- Use G-spot stimulation.

- Don't hold back when you feel the urge to urinate. Bear down.

Men either love the squirting, or they don't. There's no middle ground.

....

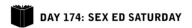 **DAY 174: SEX ED SATURDAY**

Japanese Sex #2: Shunga Sexuality

Pornography plays a significant role in modern Japanese culture. Men sometimes read graphic porn novels in the open on the subway. Love hotels include rooms designed to look like bordellos or set up to facilitate kinky sex experiences. The preference for unrestrained sexual imagery is rooted in ancient Japanese sexuality. Sex aides were easily available, with royal ladies showing off their expensive double dildos and ben wa balls at court.

Shunga sexuality gets its name from Shunga prints, in which the lovers remained clothed with only their exaggerated genitals exposed. Vulvas gaped open, dripping juice into a thicket of pubic hair; penises were massive and engorged. Get into the Shunga spirit and make sex all about your genitals today:

• Arrange your silky robes so there are openings for genitals and breasts.

• If you shave, wax, or trim pubic hair, make sure it has that fresh-from-the-salon look. If you have natural pubic hair, rub scented oil into it.

• Agree that you are free to touch, caress, fondle, and stimulate one another's genitals as long as they remain exposed.

• Set aside time that you designate for "Oral Sex on Demand," with the demand being to perform, not receive.

• Do some drawings of one another's genitals. Even if you have little or no artistic talent, a penis and a vulva are easy to draw.

············

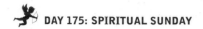 **DAY 175: SPIRITUAL SUNDAY**

Expanded Orgasm, Lesson #2

Start with a cool shower, then move to intercourse before he has an erection and build the long orgasm together.

Bodies cool from the shower, lie down facing one another in the X position, connecting only at the genitals. Her legs are between his so that she has his penis firmly between her thighs.

Holding the base of his penis in her hand, she inserts his flaccid member into her vagina. She flexes her PC muscle around it.

Synchronize your breathing. Move slowly. Stroke one another's faces, arms, breasts, and chest. Tease nipples.

Kiss deeply with eyes open.

As you move your bodies, stroke each other upward from the genitals. Imagine that you are spreading fire throughout your bodies.

Continue moving slowly in this position until you both avidly desire more vigorous thrusting. Move into another position—and go for it.

The unexpected dividend: a long, slow arousal period leads to orgasms that seem to expand from the genitals throughout the body.

....

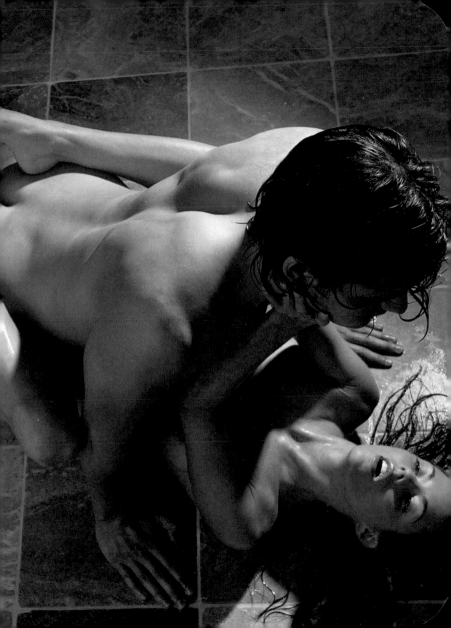

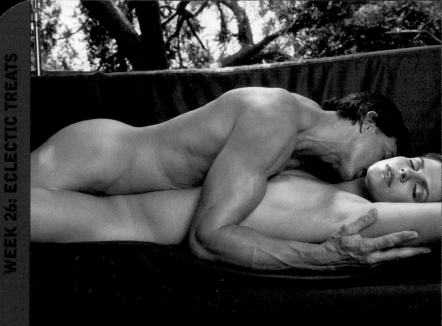

DAY 176: FLIRTATION AND FOREPLAY MONDAY

Lick an Armpit

Might armpits be the next "undiscovered erotic zone"? Admittedly, they don't get much attention in lovemaking (or daily life) unless you happen to bump up beneath one. Surprise your lover by setting your erotic sights on his (or her) armpit today.

Post-shower and pre-deodorant, put your arms around your man (or woman), hug him, and rub your nose in his chest hair or across his nipples. Then go for it: raise his arm and lick his armpit, from top to bottom, using a broad, flat tongue.

....

The Blindfolded Quickie

There are two ways of doing the Blindfolded Quickie: for the pleasure of the partner who can't see OR for the selfish satisfaction of the one in charge. If one partner really wants sex and the other is willing to give it up but doesn't want to get too involved, this is the quickie for both.

She can:

- Sit him in a chair, blindfold him, fellate him as foreplay, and sit in his lap.

- Put him on his back, tie his wrists to the headboard, blindfold him, and tease his nipples while she rides him.

- Give him a hand job or a BJ quickie.

He can:

- Tie her wrists to the bed, blindfold her, and give her a cunnilingus quickie.

- Take her rear-entry fashion using both a dildo and a vibrator on her clitoris.

- Give her a hand job quickie.

Not in the mood *and* too tired? Hand your lover the blindfold and say, "Do with me what you will . . ." Advice for the male selfish lover: Use lube. For the female: If he can't get an erection, guide his hands and mouth and give him specific directions, one step at a time.

. . . .

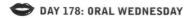 **DAY 178: ORAL WEDNESDAY**

The White House BJ Trick

Rumor has it that an intern in a previous administration tempted her president by leaving a tin of Altoids out on her desk. Apparently, he liked the curiously strong but refreshing tingle of a minty BJ. You can try this at home.

Put an Altoid in your mouth and kiss him on the mouth.

Ask him if he'd like to feel that tingling sensation in his penis.

Finish the mint before you fellate him, unless you have a particularly adept tongue (like those women who can tie a cherry stem with theirs).

If he likes the sensation, keep an Altoid box in your dresser drawer and pull it out when you want to offer him a special treat.

....

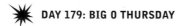 **DAY 179: BIG O THURSDAY**

His Second Coming

Men don't come again as often or as easily as women do (or at least can). But some men do have multiple orgasms. Using Taoist techniques like the ones on page 74, they have trained themselves to experience the contractions of orgasm without ejaculating. Other men (mostly young men under thirty) have short refractory periods and can reach orgasm two or more times in a lovemaking session. But some older men are capable of coming again because they work out regularly. It's all about blood flow to the cock.

Men also tell me that a partner capable of exciting them to a high level is all they need to come again. Here are some ways to encourage his second coming.

Physical Trick

After his orgasm, shift the erotic attention completely to her. Satisfy her orally and manually. Her arousal and continued orgasms will be more exciting to him than anything she can do to give him an immediate erection.

Mental Trick

Sometimes it's not about "the relationship." Learn how to separate sex from The Relationship and be carnal with one another, regardless of who hasn't done whose chores. How many sex behavior surveys have told us that women prefer shopping to sex and men would rather watch TV? People do grow too "sure" of one another. They think there are no surprises to be found in the well-known person. That's just not true. This book gives you a new idea for surprising (and delighting) each other every day.

. . . .

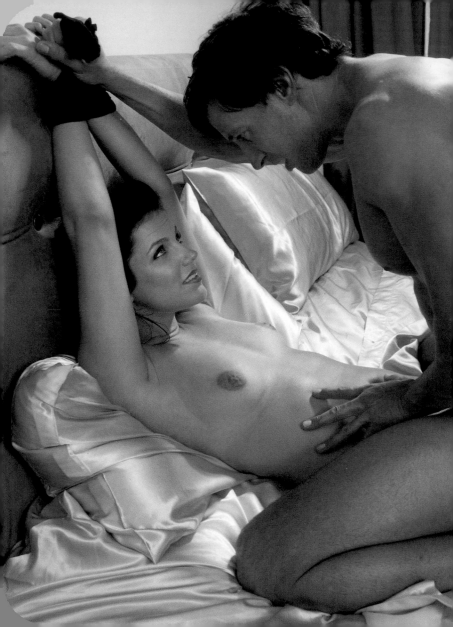

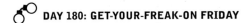 **DAY 180: GET-YOUR-FREAK-ON FRIDAY**

Tie and Tease

Even if bondage isn't on your list of preferred sex activities, you'll enjoy this playful game. It's especially nice when one partner is feeling lazy and the other is energetic. Use silk scarves or ties and don't make hard knots. The bound partner should be able to work his or her hands free easily.

If she is tied, try these tips:

- Tease her breasts and nipples with your mouth and hands.

- Run a feather up and down her torso and along her inner thighs as you lick at her labia. Use flower petals, oils and creams, and fabrics to vary the sensations as you stroke her body.

- Employ her favorite strokes on her clitoris—but only enough to arouse, not satisfy her.

- Vary the pattern of teasing by kissing her lips, then working down her body to her clit again.

- When she is begging for release, you can bring her to orgasm orally, manually, or through intercourse.

....

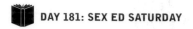

DAY 181: SEX ED SATURDAY

Modifying Your Signature Sex Move

Add a new twist to the standard routine by modifying your signature sex move, the one you perfected on page 26. The best lovers know how to change it up every now and then. If you don't, your partner is lulled into complacency. Eventually, your move might even stop working, and we can't have that!

Some suggestions:

- Is the French kiss your move? Pull back in the middle of it. Return to flirting with her lips, one at a time, with the tip of your tongue. Or kiss her breasts instead of her mouth.

- Is the BJ your special talent? Use your sucking move on his testicles instead of the head of the penis. Replace your swirling move around the head with rapid sideways flicking of the corona.

- Is cunnilingus your specialty? Leave on her wispy silk panties and suck her through the cloth. Use the tip of your chin in place of your tongue. Massage her labia with rose petals as foreplay.

....

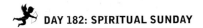 **DAY 182: SPIRITUAL SUNDAY**

Slow Sex: Stop/Start Thrusting

The easy way of prolonging lovemaking is alternating stimuli—switching from intercourse to oral or manual sex and back again. It's a particularly effective way of bringing her arousal level up to his. In Stop/Start Thrusting, intercourse is prolonged.

This classic Western sex therapy technique has its roots in both Taoist and Tantra traditions that encourage the prolonging of male arousal to accommodate his partner's slower pace. He stops thrusting when he is highly aroused, but he doesn't remove his penis from her vagina. Remaining still, he continues to pleasure her manually (or with a vibe). When his arousal level subsides but before he loses his erection, he thrusts again.

He repeats the process—stopping intercourse, starting again, manually stroking her—until she is on the verge of orgasm. Then he thrusts vigorously.

Many men report stronger orgasms after using this technique.

. . . .

DAY 183: FLIRTATION AND FOREPLAY MONDAY

Sex Journal

Buy two blank journals, his and hers. In book and specialty gift shops, you can find beautiful fabric-covered journals for less than twenty dollars and leather-bound versions for less than fifty. Or buy blank books and create your own covers. This is the modern couple's version of the Pillow Books you started some weeks ago—less art, more technique.

Some suggestions for journaling:

- Write about your sexual encounters in graphic detail.

- Paste in reviews of sexy books, recipes for special meals, and clippings of erotic stories or sex articles.

- Add sketches and drawings of favorite positions and practices if you have artistic talent, or collect erotic postcards and paste them in.

....

Her Quickie Kit

If you travel together with your partner often or have opportunities for quickies at his office or yours (or in the restroom of your favorite pub), then you need a Quickie Kit. A kit is useful even if you indulge in quickies only at home. Why waste precious minutes pulling together your sex essentials when you can have them all in one lovely little place?

Either buy a cosmetic bag or use one that came as a gift with a department store cosmetic purchase. (Lancôme gives away the best small bags.)

Now go to Babeland or another sex toy store or website and buy:

- Individual packets of lube

- Disposable cock rings

- Small vibes—finger vibes like a bullet vibe, a Pocket Rocket, or a lipstick vibe

- Condoms in individual packets and varying sizes (if you are not monogamous)

- Condoms with special features such as ribs (even if you are monogamous)

- Individually packaged wipes for cleanup

- A feather, just for fun

....

Tongue Writing on Her

This tip comes from a regular reader of my blog, SexyPrime. He is a man who loves women—and he has great sex tips.

Most guys know that "writing" on or around her clitoris is a fun game—but do they go further than spelling out a few letters?

I was really in love with a girl—and in love with her pussy—and I drew a heart around her clit. She got it right away. I created the Heart-Shaped Cunnilingus Technique for her.

Using the tip of your tongue, draw a heart around her clitoris. Repeat the move a few times.

Tell her, "Cupid is shooting arrows." Run your tongue up from her inner labia to her clitoris, flicking it with the tip of your tongue when the arrow lands. Repeat the move a few times.

Write "I love you" on the sides of her clitoris. Get your oral game on.

....

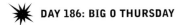 **DAY 186: BIG O THURSDAY**

The Science of Orgasm

Sex research tends to be sexist, with studies of women still focused on where orgasms come from—the clitoris, the G-spot/vagina, or both. We know more about male sexuality than female. Even given the fact that women's sex organs are tucked inside while men's are out there for scientists to measure, study, and prod into action with little blue pills, isn't this confusion over a spot inside the vagina growing ever more ridiculous?

In January 2010, British researchers announced the G-spot was either fictitious or subjective. A few weeks later, a thousand French gynecologists at a conference on the G-spot decided that the English should look harder for the illusive spot.

Do your own research study and discover whether you are one of those women claiming a G-spot. If you have a responsive G-spot, play with it.

There are three ways to find it:

1. Insert two fingers of your hand or your lover's, palm up, into your vagina, and making the tickling, "come hither" stroke. (See page 66.)

2. Experiment with a G-spot vibrator.

3. Find a penis of at least medium size that has a slight curve.

To keep up with the latest news in the science of sex, read SexyPrime. I will deconstruct the studies reported in the media for you.

. . . .

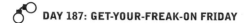 **DAY 187: GET-YOUR-FREAK-ON FRIDAY**

Honey Dust

I LOVE Honey Dust!

Made by Kama Sutra (the manufacturer, not the Indian book), Honey Dust Body Powder is a silky, delicately fragrant treat for both lovers. It is the most kissable, sensuous, edible product in the sex marketplace, and there is no shortage of powders, gels, oils, and waxy chocolate spreads designed for body licking.

Order it online or buy at a sex toy shop (or Duane Reade). New flavors include Sweet Honeysuckle, Raspberry Kiss, Strawberries & Champagne, and Tangerine & Cream.

Lightly dust your lover's lips, neck, and breasts (chest). Slowly lick and kiss the honeyed trail.

Have your lover close his or her eyes or put on a blindfold. Dust unexpected spots, such as the belly button, toes, back of the knees, and nose. Lick and suck.

Use sparingly on genitals. If you don't lick it all off, remaining bits of the product can lead to a urinary tract infection.

. . . .

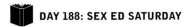

DAY 188: SEX ED SATURDAY

Advanced Chinese Sex #1:
The Tiger in the Forest Position

The authors of the Pillow Books continually reminded the male reader that women need more time in foreplay to become aroused than men do. Generally, the men took the lead in sex (and in reading, as fewer women were taught how to read). They did not move on to intercourse until they had sufficiently aroused their lovers. Only when a man had successfully courted the Jade Step (the clitoris) could he move into the Jade Pavilion (the vagina).

The Tiger in the Forest Position is a variation on rear entry designed to slow down the man's vigorous thrusting, giving the woman more time to reach orgasm.

1. She gets down on all fours on the bed, but slides her knees so that her ass is not highly elevated in the air.

2. He kneels behind her, straddles her lower legs, and fits his knees one on either side of her body.

3. His body remains upright, his hands on her ass. She has free hands to stimulate her clitoris and nipples.

....

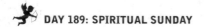

Special Orgasm Experiences:
The Soul Triggers

Many people who experience whole-body, extended, expanded, or extra-genital orgasms describe them as unique sensory experiences. Some reports from the orgasm front:

"I had tremors all over my body and I saw everything in flashing bright primary colors."

"My breasts and nipples and vaginal walls seemed to be expanding."

"It's a transcendental experience that lifts me out of my body and puts me back in again."

How do you get to that place?

- Sustained periods of arousal

- Alternating stimuli to create higher levels of arousal

- Breathing, focusing energy, eye gazing, and imaging techniques

- And the wild card—intense connection with your partner on three levels: emotional, sensual, and sexual

You can learn the techniques, but can you learn how to make those connections? Maybe they aren't skills that can be taught in the conventional way. But you are more likely to make it happen if you have good technique that leads to good sex and orgasms. Sex opens the doors to connection.

....

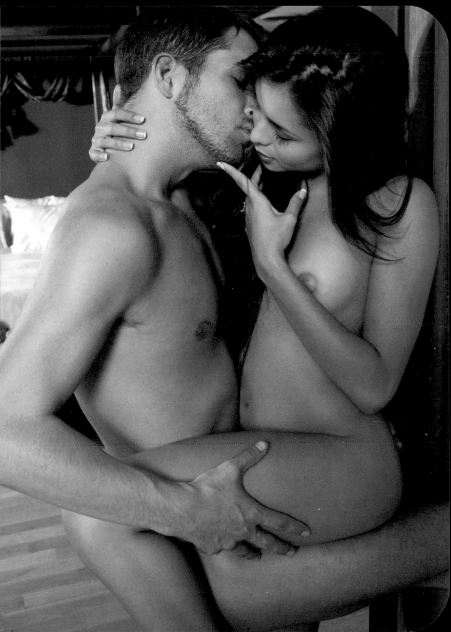

Simply Irresistible

Didn't you feel "simply irresistible" in the early days of your love affair? You couldn't keep your hands off one another. He got an erection just looking at her naked. Her nipples were always hard. And the sex . . .

Even the hottest couples reach that point (after eighteen months to three years) where the intensity of desire subsides. The body has become habituated to the love drugs created in the brain. You can manipulate it to get drunk on love again, at least for short periods of time. Sometimes the simple tricks work best.

Hold on to the hug or kiss a few beats longer than necessary, look into your lover's eyes, and say, "You are still simply irresistible."

. . . .

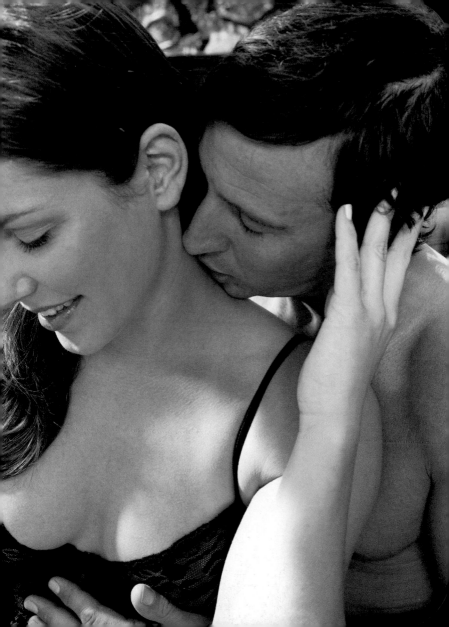

How to Seize the Moment

Quickies don't just happen. One or both lovers seize the moment. They send the little messages that say, "I want you" and "Let's do it now." Some suggestions for doing that:

- The lowered chin/raised eye look: Dip your chin a little. Now look up at your man, make eye contact, smile, and say, "I want you."

- The focused attention: When you talk to your partner, engage fully. Don't let your eyes wander. Make her feel there is no one more interesting than she is—and no place you'd rather be than naked in bed with her.

- Eye play: From across a crowded room, at a restaurant table, or over the kids' heads as you're tucking them in, look into his eyes, think a mischievous thought, and telegraph it.

- The light touch: Touch her hand or arm to emphasize a point in conversation. Brush against her and smile.

- Ask a provocative question, such as, "Would you rather I sucked your cock or begged you to fuck me?"

....

The Historical BJ #4:
Josephine's Napoleonic Treat

Emperor Napoleon and his wife Josephine documented their tempestuous sex life in hundreds of letters written to one another. They were clearly into oral sex. Some historians believe that he ultimately divorced her because she extended her oral favors to others. We also know Napoleon was an aficionado of natural body odor because he wrote Josephine, "I'm coming home—don't bathe tonight."

She was rumored to reward his victories by performing the deep throat move. We can only guess at how Josephine might have performed a Napoleonic BJ, but I think it went like this:

Wearing a long gown with your breasts popping out of the top, recline on a chaise lounge (or recliner or sofa). Ask him to thrust it between your breasts.

After a few thrusts, swirl your tongue around the head on the forward strokes. Take his cock in your hands and lightly suck the head.

Alternate sucking and swirling with long laps of the underside of your tongue up and down the shaft. Caress his balls as you strum the frenulum, flick your tongue across the corona, and swirl and suck the head.

When he is ready to come, throw your head back off the chaise and let him come down your throat, or take his cock out of your mouth and let him come on your breasts.

. . . .

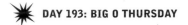 **DAY 193: BIG O THURSDAY**

Her Multiple Os #3: Serial

You read about compounded single orgasms on page 71 and sequential multiples on page 207. The difference between each of the four types—including serial and blended multiples, which follows on page 240—is largely measured in how far apart they are and how much (or whether) arousal subsides between orgasms.

Serial orgasms are multiples separated by seconds, or up to two or three minutes, with no, or barely any, interruption in stimulation or diminishment of arousal. You are most likely to encourage serial orgasms by:

- Continued and slightly varying oral stimulation, using strokes such as the Flame (page 207); the Flick, using the tip of your tongue to flick lightly and rapidly back and forth across the top of the clitoral shaft; and the Velvet "No" (page 26)

- Continued and varying manual stimulation

- Moving to intercourse after her first (oral) orgasm and adding manual stimulation as you thrust

....

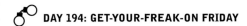 **DAY 194: GET-YOUR-FREAK-ON FRIDAY**

Fingering the Anus

If she isn't ready for anal intercourse but does enjoy a little anal play, introduce one lubed finger (or two) inside her anus during foreplay or intercourse. A good intercourse position for this is the side-by-side and face-to-face.

She puts her top leg over his top leg, opening up her anus for easy access.

He caresses her buttocks, squeezing them lightly and occasionally slapping them as he uses his other hand to stroke her clitoris.

When she's highly aroused, he inserts one lubed finger into her anus. (He wears finger cots on his anal play fingers.) These little plastic gloves for your fingertips seem less intrusive than full gloves.

Remember: Never take a finger out of her ass and put it into her pussy. This spreads bacteria.

....

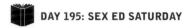

Advanced Chinese Sex #2:
Cicadas Mating

Do you have a full-length standing mirror that you can place beside the bed? This position is so beautiful—like body sculpture in motion.

She lies facedown on the bed. Supporting herself on her arms, she arches her back and raises her head, looking to the ceiling. She adjusts her legs so that they are open, one forward, knee bent at hip level, the other leg straight and angled to the side. Now she pushes her buttocks up. (She has good leverage in this position.)

He fits his body over and against hers, putting his legs between hers. He supports his weight on one arm. As he enters her from behind, he puts the other arm around her body, clasping her genitals.

As he thrusts, he strokes her labia with two fingers and massages her clitoris with his thumb.

. . . .

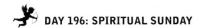 **DAY 196: SPIRITUAL SUNDAY**

Face-to-Face Position #1:
The Closer Missionary

She feels submissive; he feels, powerful. They are connected from genitals to hearts, while making deep eye contact. They may be able to sustain this slow and soulful intercourse position only for short intervals, but it will have a deep impact on both partners.

She lies on her back. He lies flat out on top of her with his pelvis a little higher than her clitoris. Once he has aligned his body to hers, he pulls up his knees to the point where he can support his weight on knees and elbows (at the sides of her chest), but he remains very tight against her.

Her arms are over her head. He holds her hands if he can do that and still balance his weight on his elbows. If not, he holds her wrists or forearms. She wraps her legs around his thighs, resting her ankles on his calves.

As they maintain deep eye contact, she leads on the upstroke, pushing her clitoris against the shaft of his penis. He leads on the downstroke, pressing the base of his penis against her clitoris.

. . . .

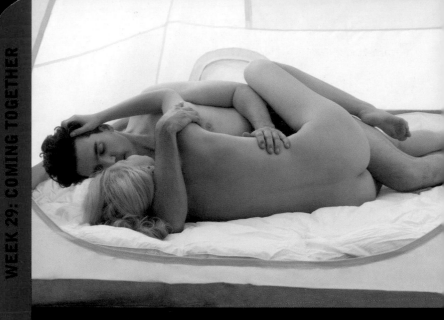

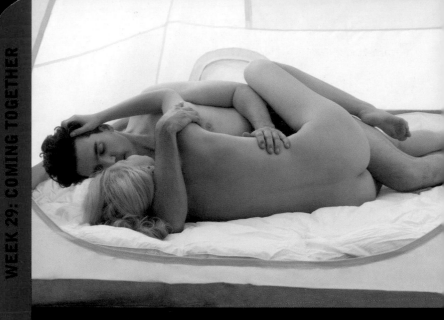 **DAY 197: FLIRTATION AND FOREPLAY MONDAY**

The Snooze Alarm Cuddle

Set the alarm for fifteen minutes earlier than usual. Hit snooze when it goes off and take your baby in your arms.

Cuddle and snooze.

Cuddle and snooze.

Isn't this a great way to start the day?

....

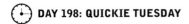

The Call Girl Special

Call girls get more requests for blow jobs than intercourse. (In some urban areas, kinky sex comes in ahead of intercourse, which is number three.) Play the call girl tonight and "service" him. Put a trench coat over your garter belt, stockings, heels, and bra—and go get the job done.

He orders the no-nonsense special. You remove your coat. He unzips his pants and pulls out his erection. You go to your knees.

Grasp the base of his penis firmly in one hand. Using the classic "loose fist" grip, slide the other hand up and down his penis. Close it when you reach the head. Repeat, repeat, repeat.

Suck his penis, primarily the head and first third of his shaft. Slide it in and out of your mouth as you work your "fist" up and down the shaft following your mouth. Repeat, repeat, repeat.

When you feel his ejaculation just beginning, take his penis out of your mouth. Slap it on your tongue in a light tapping motion. His semen will spurt out of the sides of your mouth, and he will feel like a powerful man.

....

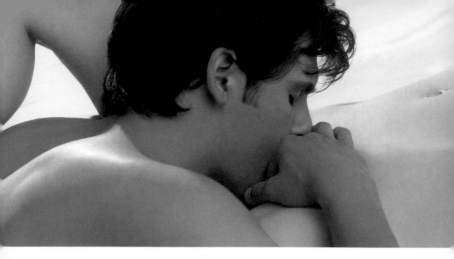

 DAY 199: ORAL WEDNESDAY

The Figure-Eight Lick, Hers

You've got your cunnilingus routine down, and it's working. That's why you need to add some new moves. In sex, once something works well and predictably, boredom looms. Total predictability is a desire killer.

This little move is simple and fun.

Using the tip of your tongue, trace a figure eight in the area surrounding her clitoris, with the clitoris itself being at the center of the 8. Repeat several times.

Now make the figure eight fancier by licking up and down the shaft in the middle of the move.

Alternate the figure eight with other moves.

....

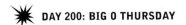 **DAY 200: BIG O THURSDAY**

The New Rear Entry: Chest Flat

Contrary to conventional wisdom, the rear-entry position is nearly as popular with women as it is with men. Women don't always want face-to-face intimacy either. Her access to her clitoris is unfettered. What is not to like?

In this version, I tweaked the angle of her upper body, which makes a difference in the sensations each lover feels. This steeper angle elongates the vagina, creating a tighter fit for his penis. (Another plus: One tester told me that having her nipple rings pressed into the mattress "stimulated my nipples like crazy.")

1. She kneels on the edge of the bed and flattens her upper body against the mattress. Her back is angled steeply down and her buttocks are raised higher.

2. He stands behind her. Clasping her buttocks, he has more thrusting freedom than in any other position.

3. If she wants him to slow down, she can use this hands-on move: Slide one hand between their bodies. Form a V with her fingers on either side of his penis. Squeeze his penis to tell him "not so hard."

....

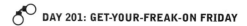

DAY 201: GET-YOUR-FREAK-ON FRIDAY

Anal Toys, His and Hers

Former porn star, director/producer, author, and entrepreneur Nina Hartley warns people that they can't expect to re-create their favorite anal sex video without a lot of lube and patience, vibes, and butt plugs. (Don't buy anything without a flared base to keep it from going where you do not want it to go.) The anus is not self-lubricating and it was not, strictly speaking, designed for intercourse. After making sure it's clean, lube and gently prepare it.

Anal Vibes

These are smaller—more slender and not as long—as vibes designed for insertion in the vagina. Work with the sphincter muscle by slowly circling with the vibe. Go slow until it opens. Then thrust gently.

Butt Plugs

These come in graduated sizes and gently open up the anus for play. Start small. They are made of softer materials, including silicone, than vibes are. Diamond-shaped and tapered for easy insertion, butt plugs are the secret prop you don't see in porn flicks, because the actress takes hers out before the scene is shot. You can buy vibrating butt plugs as well.

Anal Beads

These are strings of beads in various sizes, meant to be inserted into the anus and then gradually pulled out, creating interesting sensations.

Buy sex toys from a trusted sex toy shop or online business. I love Babeland, but also trust Good Vibrations, Booty Parlor, and some others.

If you want your lover to participate in anal intercourse, invest in the toys and give her (or him) time to discover the joys of butt play before introducing the penis or the strap-on dildo. And of course, never force anything into the anus.

....

 DAY 202: SEX ED SATURDAY

Advanced Chinese Sex #3:
The Dragon in Flight

The ancient Chinese had an aesthetic erotic sensibility that set them apart from other Eastern cultures. As you study Arabian, Indian, Chinese, and Japanese sexual arts, do you see how each has its own character in addition to its own variations on the basic positions and common practices? In the Chinese intercourse positions, the bodies come together to resemble a fanciful sculpture—in this case, a dragon in flight.

This variation of the missionary position affords her one of the best opportunities for clitoral stimulation she's likely ever known while lying on her back.

1. She lies on her back with her legs open.

(continued on next page)

2. He kneels between her legs, lifts them up, and puts them over his shoulders as he fits his body down over her. He seems to be almost prostrate in worship of her body.

The position inhibits his ability to thrust vigorously, but she can also influence their movements by using her thighs.

....

 DAY 203: SPIRITUAL SUNDAY

Simultaneous Orgasm, Lesson #1

In your grandmother's day, simultaneous orgasm was ideal. Because these spontaneous mutual combustions rarely happened for lovers who were little educated on clitoral stimulation, they were often faked. The women's revolution gave us the "ladies first" orgasm via cunnilingus (and then he had his in intercourse).

Interestingly, the simultaneous orgasm still held sway in novels and mainstream movies. Many women secretly crave the experience. Some couples strive for it. If you want to make it happen, you probably can, but timing is crucial.

1. Time how long it takes him to move from arousal to orgasm. Now time her. Dr. Joel Block has it right when he says for most couples it's an eleven-minute differential.

2. Hang on to your time cards. You will need them for lesson #2 (page 258).

....

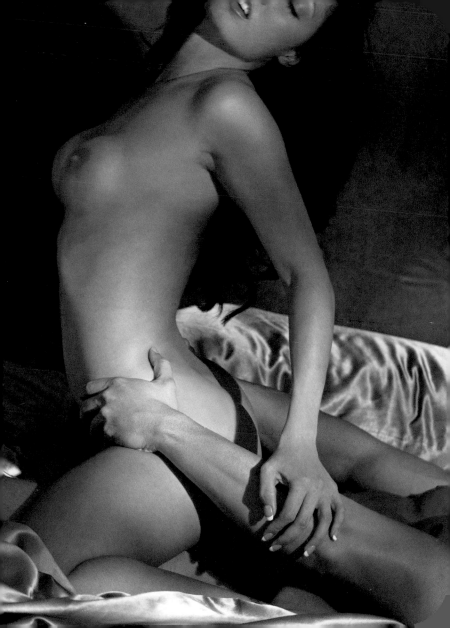

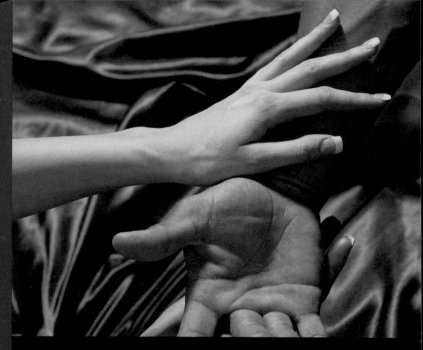

DAY 204: FLIRTATION AND FOREPLAY MONDAY

The Palm Kiss

You can do this anywhere, including in front of the kids. Yet it feels surprisingly intimate.

Hold her hand. Run your finger or thumb across her palm. Squeeze her hand. Make eye contact. Rub her palm again.

Lift her hand to your lips. Turn it over and kiss her palm as you look into her eyes.

....

The Gigolo's Delight Quickie

Traditionally, gigolos have been the masters of slow sex. Their occupation was pleasing women. They had no need to rush off. The women they pleased were wealthy and unemployed. The modern gigolo spends a lot of time in the gym to maintain the look women will buy, and the women who buy have careers.

This quickie is from Michel, French gigolo par excellence.

The mood is everything. She doesn't have time to see you, but you must see her. You must have her. She consents. You arrive at her office or home in a state of high sexual agitation. You sweep her into your arms and take her.

Shower her face, neck, throat, and cleavage with hot, passionate kisses as you run your hands hungrily over her body.

Firmly caress her buttocks and pull her to you while kissing her deeply.

Unzip your pants with one hand and push her panties aside with the other.

Push her up against a wall or bend her over a piece of furniture—and take her.

Her orgasm is beside the point. She will masturbate later to the memory of your need for her, so great it could not be denied. Michel says, "Every woman needs to be taken like this occasionally. It reminds her of who she is, a woman who can drive a man out of his mind with desire."

. . . .

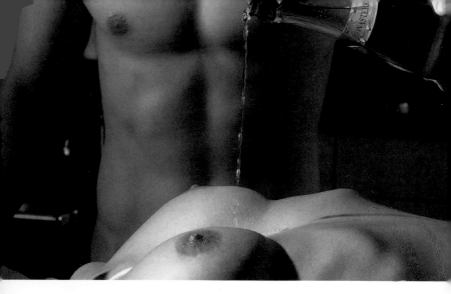

 DAY 206: ORAL WEDNESDAY

The French Tickler, Hers

Pop the cork on a chilled bottle of champagne. Put it in an ice bucket and take it with you to bed.

Before going down on her, take a swig of champagne.

Hold it in your mouth until your lips touch her clit. Open them slightly to let a little champagne out.

Swirl the bubbles around her clit with your tongue, letting a few drops of champagne out with each movement.

The bubbles will heighten the sensations of oral sex for her.

....

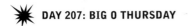 **DAY 207: BIG O THURSDAY**

The New Sitting Position:
Backward Lean

In the Reverse Cowgirl position, you ride him facing his feet, not his head. You probably sit almost straight or lean forward slightly. This variation is a bit challenging, but the reward is greater G-spot stimulation.

Straddle him, facing his feet. Rise up on your toes, your heels at his buttocks, so that your legs are bent like chicken wings.

Place your hands on his forearms and lean backward. Arch your back and turn your face up.

He puts his hands on your hips to help steady you and guide thrusting.

As you thrust, feel the extra stimulation on your G-spot.

. . . .

 DAY 208: GET-YOUR-FREAK-ON FRIDAY

Anal Intercourse: The Basics

If everything you know about anal sex you learned from watching porn, then you need new learning. In real life, you don't just roll a woman over and slip it in. They don't do it that way in porn either. Before the shoot, the actress has had an enema or three, worn a butt plug, and injected syringes of lube up her anus.

Anal intercourse can be thrilling for her as well as him, but only if it's done right.

Here are the basics:

- Lube, lube, lube! The anus is not the vagina. It does not self-lubricate.

- Anal condoms, disposable plastic gloves, or finger cots. Bacteria that live in the anus can give him and her a urinary tract infection— or worse.

- Preparation. She needs to be highly aroused. Pull out all the foreplay stops. Use your best oral and manual moves. Insert first one lubricated and gloved finger into her anus, then add another finger.

- When she is ready, penetrate her slowly. Don't force your way past the sphincter muscle. Help her relax it by stroking her clitoris (with a clean hand). Let her control the speed and depth of entry by pushing against you.

- Don't thrust vigorously the way you've seen it done in porn. (Do you know that many of those actresses have required anal repair surgeries?) Follow her lead on how deep and how fast.

....

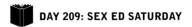

Puritan Sex #2: The White Nightgown

Buy a deceptively sexy white nightgown. Let wearing it be your signal to him that you want to be taken in haste and darkness like a Puritan wife.

The Setup

Hester Prynne, forced to wear the scarlet A for adultery in Nathaniel Hawthorne's *The Scarlet Letter,* is your role model. She seethed with passion for her minister/lover Arthur Dimmesdale. You can't help yourself. Tonight, you will sin again.

But, unlike poor Hester, you have a wardrobe of vibes to ensure that you will be at the point of orgasm when you put on the nightgown and announce your desire to your man.

The Position

Missionary—what else?!

Hike up your nightgown, and do it under the sheets with the lights off. And no talking, please.

An occasional down-and-dirty fuck is a good thing, yes? (It's even better because you don't live in the seventeenth century and don't have to do it this way every time.)

....

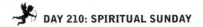

Simultaneous Orgasm, Lesson #2

There's only one place to make up the critical time difference: foreplay. The faster partner (almost certainly him) focuses more oral and manual attention on the "slower" partner (most likely her). Don't begin intercourse until the two of you are in sync.

She keeps one hand on his back or thigh to communicate her readiness to move on.

He knows the signs of high arousal—sweating, panting, trembling thighs, shaky voice, splotchy chest. Watch for them. Keep up the stimulation until you see them. Maintaining eye contact will also help. Check your time cards so you will know how long this takes for each partner.

. . . .

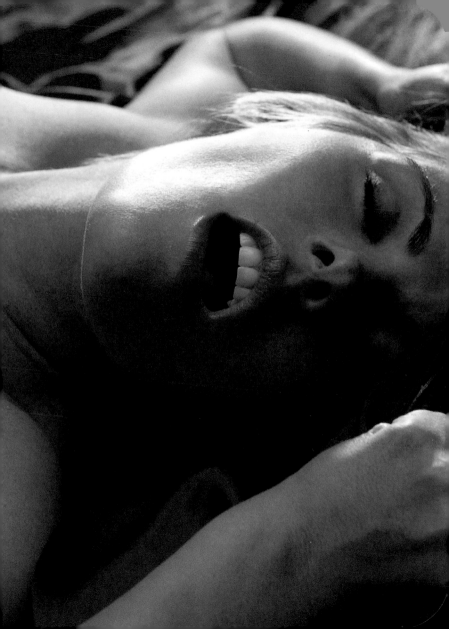

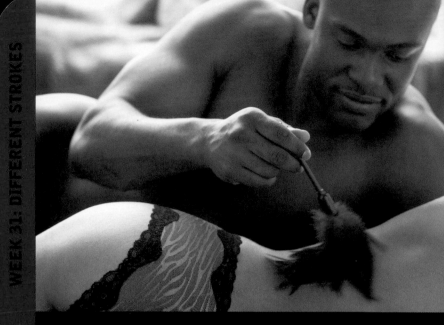

DAY 211: FLIRTATION AND FOREPLAY MONDAY

Hand/Arm Strokes #1: Feathers

Is there a more erotically neglected body part than arms? We use them to hug and they power many sexual activities, but do they get a share of the love?

Pull out your favorite feather. Run it up and down your lover's bare arm. Tickle the armpits. Take his hand in yours and brush the feather across his wrist. Tickle his palm. Repeat with the other arm and hand.

The soft touch of a feather stirs our skin.

....

Head of the Penis Quickie Trick

Can you slow down intercourse and still call it a quickie? Yes, if the slowdown only lasts a minute or two. That may be all she needs to get her orgasm, too. Woman on top (female superior) is the best position for pulling this off.

She pulls up so that only the tip of the head of his penis is inserted in her vagina.

While playing with her clit, she lowers herself onto the head and pulls back up. (The teasing drives him wild.)

When she's near orgasm, she thrusts down onto his penis, grinding her clitoris into his public bone.

....

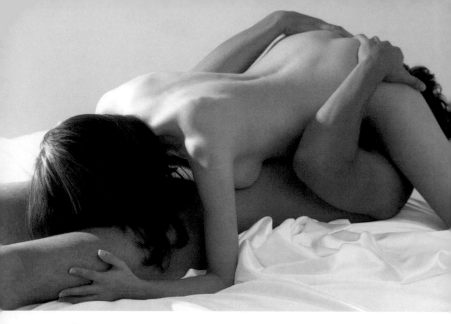

 DAY 213: ORAL WEDNESDAY

Strumming the Frenulum

The frenulum is that piece of loose skin on the underside of the shaft, below the head. It is exquisitely sensitive on some men. This very simple move may persuade him that you are an oral genius.

With the tip of your tongue, strum rapidly back and forth across the frenulum.

Pull back. Lick it in broad strokes.

Strum again.

....

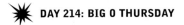 **DAY 214: BIG O THURSDAY**

Her Multiple Os #4: Blended

You learned about compounded single orgasms on page 71, sequential multiples on page 207, and serial multiples on page 240. Blended multiples are the last type of multiple orgasms women can experience. They are simply a mix of two or more of the first three types.

There is something called a blended orgasm, which is a single orgasm that results from more than one form of stimulation, such as clitoral and G-spot. Most single orgasms are probably blended. But the single blended orgasm and blended multiples are different, great moments.

Very often, women who are multiply orgasmic do experience blended multiples. You can encourage them by:

- Receiving both clitoral and vaginal stimulation at the same time

- Adding a vibrator to sex play

- Alternating intense stimuli with softer strokes, and staying on the verge of orgasm for a long time before you let yourself have the first one

....

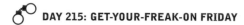

Get Your Laugh On

A slew of sex books by stand-up comics have landed on my desk in recent weeks. If you want to be really freaky, get your laugh on. Laughing about "bad sex" (and preferably not yours) is a bonding experience, just like watching a funny movie where the characters keep getting love and sex wrong. Sometimes sex is funny.

This comes from Rebecca, who looks ten years younger than her thirty-eight years, a tiny, stunning, fashion-savvy woman with that creamy cafe au lait skin—a woman who looks like she must be hot in bed. But, she says, not so much. She's blunt and bold, and she *should* be a stand-up comic.

Whatever happened to straight sex? Men want all this stuff! Anal! Coming on your face! What's wrong with your penis in my vagina? Men don't want women. They want dolls they can pose like porn stars and do whatever they want to them.

Sex isn't fun anymore. I'd rather eat Häagen-Dazs.

I don't come that often anyway.

If a guy is going for my elusive orgasm, I should tell him: We could be here all day and I have to go to work.

In my head I'm thinking about cleaning the bathroom while he's trying to get me off. I look at my feet and wonder if I'm pointing them enough. I have to keep cute poses! Then I realize that I need a pedicure.

And I've lost the possibility of orgasm.

Uh! Oh! Uh! . . . Oh, I don't think so.

. . . .

📖 **DAY 216: SEX ED SATURDAY**

Advanced Indian Sex #1:
Kneeling Man

The erotic temple carvings in India depict couples in contorted inter-course positions that sometimes look more painful than sexy. Yet the Kama Sutra includes many positions that can be adapted for comfort without changing the coital dynamics that work to speed her arousal and slow his ejaculation. This one is a clever variation of the standing posi-tion, but it gives her the thrusting power. Try it; you will like it.

1. He kneels on the floor with a wall or piece of furniture close enough on one side to give him support, if needed.

2. She kneels on one leg between his and wraps the other leg around his waist.

3. He supports her by holding the buttock of the leg wrapped around his waist.

4. She holds on to his shoulders, throws her head back, and thrusts against him.

. . . .

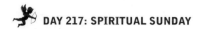

Simultaneous Orgasm, Lesson #3

Not bringing her to orgasm first is probably the most difficult part of this exercise for him. He is used to taking care of her before he takes care of himself. For the modern Western male lover, "she comes first" is a key part of the credo.

For this lesson, you'll need to abandon the "ladies first" mentality:

Get her to the brink of orgasm. Take a minute to catch up to her now because she pulled ahead of you.

Start intercourse at the same place—on high arousal.

Keep your hands on each other's hips or backs to communicate, if necessary, to slow it down.

If you got the timing right, you will come together. And if not, try again another day.

....

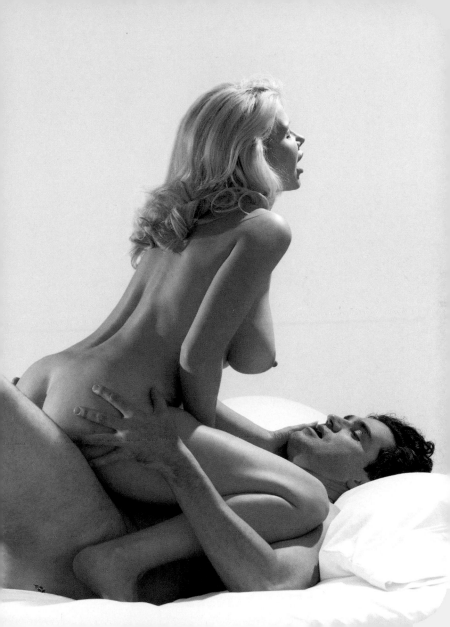

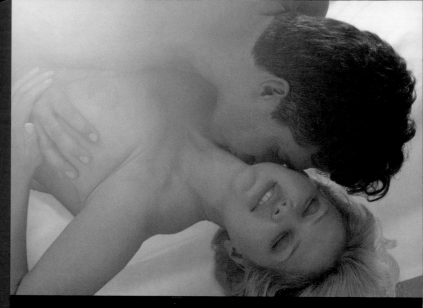

DAY 218: FLIRTATION AND FOREPLAY MONDAY

Hand/Arm Strokes #2:
Circling Fingers

You woke up those arms and hands last week with a feather. Give them a little more attention today. Having one's body caressed, however briefly and chastely, is mood elevating.

Curve the fingers of one hand. Rest them on your lover's arm. Make little circling movements with each finger pad. Move the circles up and down his arm.

Now use the same move on the other arm.

....

Bathroom Quickie #1: The Nozzle

A lot of women masturbate in the tub or shower by using the shower nozzle on their clits. Whether you have a fixed nozzle, a handheld shower nozzle, or Jacuzzi jets, take advantage of the water power to get your orgasm in a bathroom quickie.

1. As he's getting ready to shower, tell him, "I feel dirty. I'll join you."

2. Kiss and caress him as you are both pulling your clothes off.

3. Keep your hand on his penis while you adjust the water temperature.

4. In the shower, he angles his body so that his erection rubs against her labia as she soaps his chest; he pushes beneath her buttocks, again teasing her labia, as he soaps her back.

5. She adjusts the shower nozzle to spray her clitoris. He enters her from behind.

....

The Corona Lick #2

The corona, the ridge separating the head of the penis from the shaft, is one of the most sensitive places on the penis. You surely touch upon it frequently while performing fellatio. (See page 70.) Tonight make it the star receiver. Keep all the attention on his corona until he begs you to suck him.

1. Flick your tongue back and forth lightly across the corona.

2. After several flicks, run your tongue from the base to the head, swirling it around the corona.

3. Flick back and forth several times again.

4. Put your lips over the head and purse them around the corona. Suck gently.

5. Return to the flick.

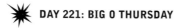

✳ DAY 221: BIG O THURSDAY

Encouraging Multiple Os

You can now identify the kinds of multiple orgasms and have learned some tips for encouraging them. Put it all together today—and come and come again. First, get rid of old attitudes that might be holding you back, like thinking you have to rush through your orgasm so he can have his.

Focus

You need to be focused on your own pleasure to have multiple orgasms. Don't worry about pleasing him. He will be excited by your multiples and possibly find them as good as his own orgasm. Men love satisfying women. Close your eyes if you need to do that to maintain your solitary focus.

Alternating Stimulation

After the first orgasm, many women are too sensitive for direct clitoral stimulation. So, her partner stops stroking her, and her arousal subsides. Drawing from a variety of oral and manual moves in other sections, he should sustain her arousal. Shift from the clitoris to the surrounding tissues or labia or G-spot.

Repeated Direct Stimulation

Some women do need the continued direct licking, suckling, stroking, or vibrating of the clitoris to come again. If you are one of those women, your obstacle to having multiples may simply be this: You (and your lover) quit too soon. Sustain arousal through one orgasm and then see what happens.

. . . .

 DAY 222: GET-YOUR-FREAK-ON FRIDAY

Anal Intercourse Positions

The three basic anal intercourse positions are rear entry, female superior, and missionary. My colleague Tristan Taormino's book, *The Anal Sex Position Guide*, has many variations on the basics—and much other good information on what works depending on your experience with anal sex, his penis size, and other factors. The receiver should control the depth and speed of penetration no matter which position they choose.

Rear Entry

This one you usually see in porn films. She gets down on all fours and he stands or kneels behind.

Advantages: He has a great view of her ass and she (or he) has easy access to her clitoris.

Potential disadvantage: He might thrust too vigorously.

Female Superior

He lies down; she straddles him and lowers herself onto his penis.

Advantage: She is in control.

Potential disadvantage: She may be so reluctant to lower herself onto him (fearing pain) that penetration takes a long time.

Missionary

She lies on her back as he kneels in front of her. She draws her knees up, putting her feet against his chest.

Advantages: She is in a good position for control.

Potential disadvantage: Some women experience the penetration as being fuller and deeper—and more uncomfortable—in this position.

....

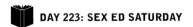

Advanced Indian Sex #2:
The Contrary Position

Thousands of years ago, India's most celebrated courtesans were adept practitioners of the female superior position. The ordinary wife might have spent more time in the missionary position than any other. But courtesans had erotic power, as did the temple priestesses, for whom sex was sacred.

What a contrast to our times, when the role of wife is elevated over that of mistress or sexually active single woman—and sex advice is aimed at monogamous couples! Western culture sanctifies and sanitizes married sex. Pretend you are an ancient courtesan in this position—and see whether desanctifying your sex life occasionally doesn't make it hotter.

1. He lies on his back.

2. She lies flat on top of him.

3. As he enters her, she arches her back and presses her hands against his chest or waist (depending on their relative heights).

4. Leveraging against his body, she thrusts her hips in a circular motion.

The position gives her both clitoral and G-spot stimulation and helps him sustain arousal longer.

....

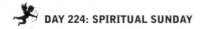

Whole-Body Orgasm

Occasionally, an orgasm is both intense and diffuse, with tremors radiating from the genitals to the body's extremities. Some people experience whole-body orgasms only when they are very connected to their partners. For others, it is a deeply personal experience facilitated by the lover.

Imagine orgasmic waves getting bigger and bigger as they wash over your body. Make it happen first during masturbation. Either take turns, with one lover watching the other, or do it simultaneously.

Her Whole-Body Orgasm

1. Masturbate in a comfortable position.

2. As soon as you become highly aroused, use your other hand to massage your vulva, inner thighs, and groin with light, shallow strokes. Imagine that you are spreading arousal throughout those areas.

3. Continue the massage during your orgasm, imagining you are spreading the orgasm into your body.

His Whole-Body Orgasm

1. You need a strong PC muscle for this. During masturbation (and later intercourse), stop thrusting when you feel ejaculation is imminent. Flex the PC muscle and hold for a count of nine. Or try flexing nine times in rapid succession instead of holding the count.

2. Now resume thrusting.

....

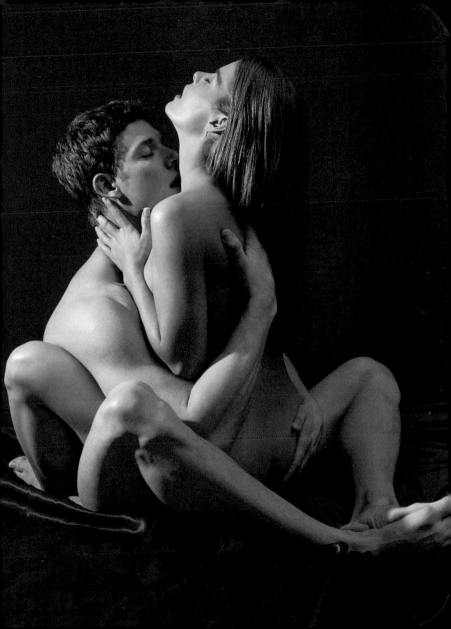

Hand/Arm Strokes #3:
Deep Pressing Fingers

Give your lover's arms a mini massage with this stroke. She will want to know those pressing fingers all over her body.

1. Rest your hand, fingers spaced comfortably apart, on your lover's arm.

2. Using your finger pads, including your thumb, press into her flesh.

3. Move your pressing fingers up and down each arm.

4. Take her hand and press your thumb against her wrist and your fingers on the back of her hand.

5. Repeat on the other arm.

. . . .

Bathroom Quickie #2:
"Put the Lid Down"

Take the sitting intercourse position to a new place: the toilet. Doing it on the toilet is both witty and naughty, with a bonus of great leverage for both of you. Depending on your heights, you might both have your feet on the ground.

Why didn't we think of this sooner?

Walk naked into the bathroom as she is toweling off from her bath or shower and offer to put some lotion on her back. Rub it into her butt, too. Turn her around and smooth lotion into her breasts, tummy, and thighs.

You have an erection. It's bouncing against her vulva. She likes what she sees.

Kiss and caress her in a standing position, pressing your penis against her but not into her.

When she suggests going into the bedroom, suggest doing it right where you are. Put down the lid and throw a towel over it. Sit down with your legs comfortably apart. Guide her down onto your erection.

She has a lot of room to maneuver; for example, she can rise up and down on her toes while you remain stationary. Or, you can thrust up and down, powered by your legs, as you rock her back and forth.

. . . .

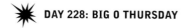

DAY 227: ORAL WEDNESDAY

The Urban BJ #1: Up on the Roof

On a balmy night, take him up on the roof. Spread a blanket out. Pour some wine. Drink a little. Lie down together. Kiss and fondle until he has a nice erection. Then unzip his pants, take out his cock, and give him a rooftop BJ.

1. Press your lips against his shaft as you caress his balls.

2. Lick your way up the shaft to the head while lightly scratching his balls.

3. Holding his penis in both hands, work your magic on the head, alternating swirling tongue strokes with gentle sucks.

4. Tongue the corona. Suck the head. Work the shaft with your hands. Bring him to orgasm in your mouth.

You want him to come relatively quickly. (Someone else might decide to use the roof.) Combining intense oral head moves with good hand action will do that.

....

DAY 228: BIG O THURSDAY

The Surprise Orgasm

You're not in the mood. Your lover is more highly aroused than you are. You're mad at him. Or, in this case, you don't know or particularly like him. But you COME—in a spectacular, fireworks-exploding kind of orgasm. What's that all about? I don't know. It defies science. But with luck, you will have one someday. Be open to the idea.

This is a story from SexyPrime:

Ben, an art dealer I know in the 'hood, introduced me to B, his friend, an artist from Senegal. B is not my type. Too old (about my age—and you know I am a cougar). Too much unfocused sexual energy (coming on to every woman in our section of the bar). Too insistent (once he focused on me, probably by default because the other babes weren't buying him). Too interested in feet (kissing and caressing my ankle and instep). Didn't like his kiss. Didn't believe he was all the things he said he was. (Googled him this morning. Wrong. He is all that. But I'm still betting he lied about being unattached. Ha!) Yet I ended up in his arms.

From there, he did almost nothing the way I wanted it done. Apparently, I wasn't pleasing him either. He kept telling me he liked that big thing deep throated. And I wasn't ready to die, suffocated by a big dick down my throat.

But a funny thing happened when he fucked me, in the more or less classic missionary position with one of my legs wrapped around his waist and the other wrapped beneath his sinewy buttock. It felt so good. It felt like coming home, if home is a place of pure erotic bliss.

I started to come. And I kept coming. And coming and coming and coming.

He woke me Sunday morning, making the case for a blow job before coffee; I didn't even argue. When he came in my mouth, he seemed to come forever, the throbbing like aftershocks I felt in my pussy.

. . . .

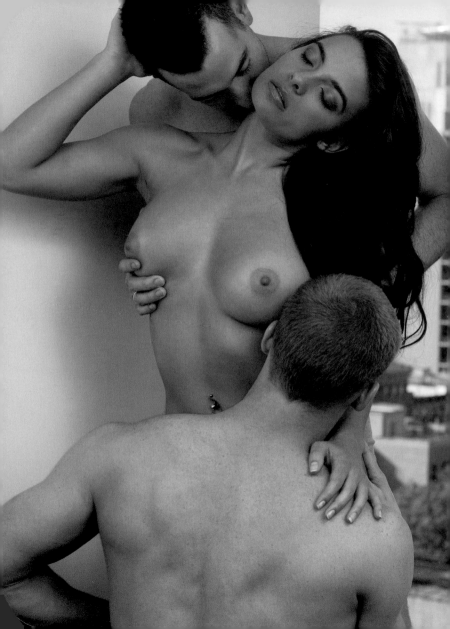

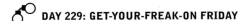 **DAY 229: GET-YOUR-FREAK-ON FRIDAY**

Create a Secret Life

The compulsion to tell one's partner everything is annoyingly American and erotically stifling. You need a private sex life. Maybe this place will exist only in your head. That's fine. Nurture your fantasy garden; you can renew, replenish, and reinvent your sexuality.

Some secret life suggestions:

- Visit a nude beach.

- Let your secret "top" or "bottom" come out—in fantasy if not reality.

- Make sexual demands.

- Go to a swing club.

- Buy a new sex toy and keep it from your lover.

- Ditto for a DVD.

- Have a flirtation (or a fling?) with someone else.

- Masturbate—and don't tell your lover.

- Go out alone for a drink and seduce a stranger.

- Tell an opposite-sex friend a sexual secret your partner doesn't know.

Make your secret sex life wish lists—and don't share them.

....

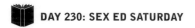

Advanced Indian Sex #3:
Splitting the Bamboo

This isn't as difficult as you think it's going to be. If you can lie on your back and do a scissors kick with your legs, then you can do this one.

1. She lies on her back with her legs open. He kneels in front of her.

2. As he enters her, he lifts her legs and places them on his shoulders.

3. She plays with her clit as he thrusts.

4. When she is very aroused, she begins to split the bamboo—stretching out one leg to the side and then the other. This slows his thrusting and prolongs both their high arousal states.

5. She signals that she is ready to thrust to climax by drawing her knees to her chest, placing her feet on his chest, and pushing against his penis.

....

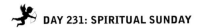 **DAY 231: SPIRITUAL SUNDAY**

How to Give Her a Whole-Body Orgasm

You watched her masturbate to a whole-body orgasm, and you've done it yourself. With her help, "give" her the whole-body experience. It's a slow, sensual ride.

The techniques you've both learned for prolonging intercourse and extending and expanding orgasm were largely unknown to Western culture until the nineteenth century, but they were practiced in other cultures for thousands of years. The ancient Polynesians, for example, believed intercourse should last an hour. The Arabs practiced *imsak*, meaning "retention," with the man pulling out when he felt close to orgasm, but continuing to stimulate his partner with his hand or mouth until he was able to resume thrusting again.

Put a little *imsak* in your intercourse today. Foreplay is for her only. Arouse her with your hands and mouth, but stop short of giving her an orgasm.

Get into a comfortable intercourse position (likely to change several times) and thrust slowly, practicing *imsak* when you are too aroused.

Alternate oral and manual moves, and bring her to orgasm once or several times, each time massaging her vulva, inner thighs, and lower belly as if you were drawing the contraction outward. Try not to reach orgasm until she is sated—and she may come one more time.

············

DAY 232: FLIRTATION AND FOREPLAY MONDAY

Rub His Chest

Men's bodies are so nice, aren't they? The chest is particularly attractive. But how often do we remember to stroke and kiss it?

Catch him with his shirt open, either in the process of dressing or undressing. Put your arms around him and bury your face in his chest. Rub your nose in his hair (if he has hair) and across his nipples.

With one hand, rub his chest. Alternate broad flat palm moves with using your finger pads to press and rub. Lightly scratch him if he likes that.

....

DAY 233: QUICKIE TUESDAY

Quickie Dressing

Is your wardrobe quickie-friendly? You need some clothes that are seductive (albeit in a classy way) and easily shed, preferably in layers. Maybe your sex date tonight should begin with a trip to the mall.

Some suggestions:

• Silk blouses

• Pencil skirts

• Wrap dresses (in the style of Diana von Furstenberg)

- Tailored slacks with front or side zippers

- Thigh-high stockings (*not* pantyhose)

- Stiletto sling-back pumps

- Minimalist jewelry

- Silk or silky-soft kimono, robes, and dressing gowns

- Beautiful matching bra and panty sets

....

👄 DAY 234: ORAL WEDNESDAY

The Urban CJ #1: Up on the Roof

It's his turn to take her up on the roof. She should wear a full skirt and no panties—cover for his busy mouth and no obstacles in his way.

Stretch out on the blanket in a full-body embrace. Kiss her the way she loves to be kissed. Put your hand under her skirt and warm up her pussy. Now go under that skirt. Gently part her labia lips. Place a finger on either side of her clitoris, and press down lightly.

Put the tip of your tongue against the shaft of her clitoris. Move your head back and forth while holding your tongue steady. You're vibrating her clitoris without a vibe!

Make little darting moves with the tip of your tongue up and down her shaft. When you get to the top, swirl the head. Repeat these moves. Add gentle sucking when she is ready to come.

....

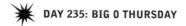 **DAY 235: BIG O THURSDAY**

Fire Up Your Orgasm

The Breath of Fire is the quickest way I know to jump-start either my sexual energy or my libido. It oxygenates the blood quickly, truly building fire. Do this before sex, either together or separately: Take rapid, rhythmic, and shallow breaths through your nose while keeping your mouth closed. Breathe this way for one to three minutes. Feel your heartbeat accelerate and your genitals respond.

Now incorporate fire breathing into intercourse in any position.

Pull your breath deeply into your body on the upstroke. Imagine that huge intake of air goes all the way into your genitals.

As you exhale on the downstroke, push the air out of your body.

After a dozen or so deep breaths on slow thrusts, pant by breathing rapidly from your belly with your mouth open as you increase the speed of thrusting.

Alternate the short breaths/fast strokes with deep breaths/slow strokes.

As you near orgasm, make the breathing a continuous circular motion.

Imagine this circle of fire going out her nose into his, down through his genitals into hers, and up again.

Your orgasms will feel like they are on fire.

....

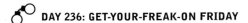 **DAY 236: GET-YOUR-FREAK-ON FRIDAY**

Meet the Strap-On

The unexpected success of the video series *Bend Over Boyfriend* has widened the market for strap-on dildos, once a toy purchased primarily by lesbians, not straight women. Some men do enjoy anal penetration and some women are willing to oblige them. And other women say to their men, "If you want me to receive anal sex, you give that position a try for a change."

The Dildo/Harness Options

You can, of course, manually use a dildo to penetrate his anus, but adding a harness frees your hands and gives you a new thrill—thrusting. The basic harness straps the dildo onto your body via adjustable straps around the waist and thighs. A two-strap harness has two leg straps that wrap around the thighs and attach to a slim waistband. The G-string harness looks like a leather thong with a single strap running up the center of the butt, attaching to a slim waistband.

A strap-on kit contains a dildo and a harness—a good choice for beginners because the kits come with instructions.

The vibrating harness is the luxury product in the category. Two little vibrating pads are attached to the harness, one next to her clitoris, the other located where the dildo comes out of the harness.

....

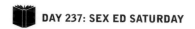**DAY 237: SEX ED SATURDAY**

The Laziest Tantra Position

Many Tantra positions appear daunting to those of us who have not been trained as gymnasts. This one is *so* easy. Consider it the sex ed equivalent of lunch, or school assemblies, or homeroom. (You aced them all, right?)

She kneels on the floor and drapes the top half of her body across a couch, table, or other surface.

He kneels, straddles her legs, and enters her from behind.

He holds on to her hips as he thrusts. Leaning forward on her forearms, she pushes back against him.

You can do this one outside the bedroom—and without removing any clothing except her panties—which makes it ideal for spontaneous sex before going out on Saturday night.

. . . .

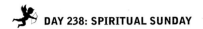 **DAY 238: SPIRITUAL SUNDAY**

How to Give Him a Whole-Body Orgasm

Most men learned in adolescence how to ejaculate as quickly as possible to avoid being caught masturbating. No wonder they are goal-oriented lovers striving to last long enough to give a woman pleasure but not expecting more than a few seconds of ejaculatory bliss for themselves. Help him take it to the limit today.

You have watched him masturbate to a whole-body orgasm. Follow that pattern. Stop when he needs to stop. You take over the hand moves that will extend his orgasm and spread it throughout his body.

Keep foreplay to a minimum for him, but let him stimulate you as much as you desire—even to orgasm.

Get into a comfortable intercourse position. You'll have more control if you're on top, but it's not essential. He keeps his hand on your thigh or buttock and communicates when he needs a pause.

He will be employing the techniques he's learned—PC flexing, *imsak*— to prolong intercourse. When he is ready to ejaculate, take his penis in hand. Continue stimulating it slowly through his orgasm. At the same time, use your other hand to massage his perineum, groin, and inner thighs.

· · · · · · · · · · · ·

DAY 239: FLIRTATION AND FOREPLAY MONDAY

Lick an Instep

A regular SexyPrime reader sent this tip:

My girlfriend and I had been arguing over her having dinner with an old boyfriend. I didn't want her to go—I was jealous—but she insisted that she would see him. They were out so late that I fell asleep (aided by a few shots of Jameson's scotch) waiting for her to come home. I did hear her come in but pretended to be asleep.

Suddenly I felt her tongue running up my instep. She licked my foot! Then she settled her body against mine and went to sleep. We had great sex in the morning.

Some tension in the bed when you slip in behind your mate? Lick his (her) instep and fit your body against his. Morning may dawn brighter than usual.

. . . .

 DAY 240: QUICKIE TUESDAY

The Red Heels Quickie

A photo on Photobucket.com inspired this quickie. The photo: a woman with great legs wearing red stiletto pumps sitting on the edge of the bed, her feet on the bare chest of a hunk in blue jeans standing before her. What woman wouldn't want some of that?

The Preparations

The red heels are a must! If you don't own a pair, buy, beg, steal, or borrow them. They set the mood so effectively that, even if you've never had sex with your shoes on, you won't see any other way to do it this time.

Put on your tiniest skirt, preferably a denim mini (but black is good, too). Add a big white shirt, unbuttoned, tied around your waist.

Tell that hunk to take off his shirt and "Come here!" But he can only watch, not touch, until you invite him to play.

The Quickie

Rest your heels on his chest and give him a good view of your naked pussy.

Hike up your skirt and play with your clitoris as you "walk" up and down his chest.

Continue stroking yourself—making uninhibited noises—as you "walk" over the bulge in his pants. After you elicit a moan from him, invite him to play.

Wrap your legs around his waist or put them over his shoulders, whichever feels right to you, and let him take you standing up.

....

The Tut-Tut Suck, Hers

Have you ever heard anyone make the "tut-tut" sound—usually accompanied by shaking the head back and forth—to indicate disapproval? (Message: You've been naughty.) The "tut-tut" sound is a clicking of the tip of the tongue. Tell your favorite clitoris how naughty she's been in a way that makes her realize you like naughty girls.

1. Put your lips around the sides of her clitoris. Hold them in a slightly pursed position.

2. Alternate light sucking with the tut-tut tip of your tongue click.

3. As you are tut-tutting, shake your head gently from side to side.

4. Switch off to your usual oral strokes, but return to the tut-tut suck moves.

....

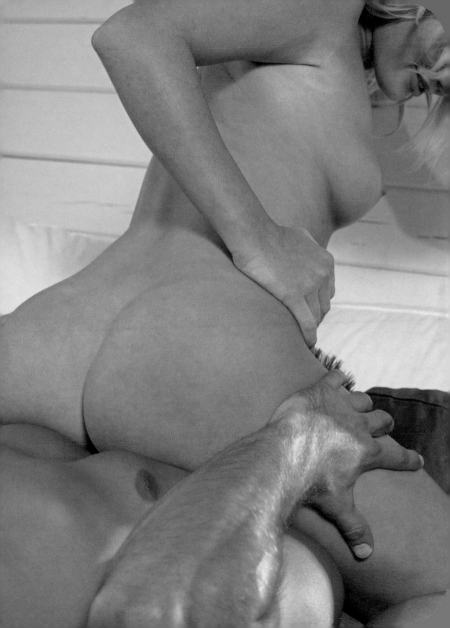

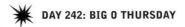 **DAY 242: BIG O THURSDAY**

Alternating Orgasms

Take turns having an orgasm and watching your lover come. You can do this as part of mutual masturbation, with oral or manual sex, or during intercourse. Both try to last as long as possible and do so by halting stimulation to let the other "catch up." The one who can't take it any longer comes first.

Take turns arousing one another. During intercourse, for example, he can stop thrusting and stroke her clitoris and suck her nipples. When she is highly aroused, he stops or slows her stimulation and thrusts again.

If they are masturbating side by side, the partner who is near orgasm stops and watches the other.

Fellatio/cunnilingus or hand jobs are handled the same way: Bring one partner close to orgasm, then switch off and stimulate the other.

It's exciting to watch your partner come. Being desperate for release yourself as you watch gives it a special edge.

....

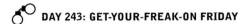 **DAY 243: GET-YOUR-FREAK-ON FRIDAY**

Strap-On Thrusting Techniques

Prepare him to receive anal sex in the same way he prepares you (see page 255). Key word: lube!

- Make sure he is aroused and well lubricated before you penetrate his anus.

- Insert the dildo slowly.

- Let him direct the depth of penetration and speed of thrusting.

- Thrust confidently, like you know what you're doing.

A SexyPrime reader wrote this about her first experience penetrating her husband:

I talked him into it. We ordered a kit online. But when I opened it, I thought: Oh, no! *He had some pangs of doubt and fear, too. We drank a little wine and said, "Oh, what the hell, let's see what this is all about."*

We were both surprised at how much we enjoyed switching roles, me thrusting, him receiving. It changed our relationship—for the better.

. . . .

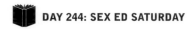 **DAY 244: SEX ED SATURDAY**

Advanced Japanese Sex #1:
The Deep Waters Rear-Entry Position

A large portion of ancient Japanese art and literature, especially the poetry, was devoted to the erotic arts. Glorious paintings and illustrations in sex books qualify as great sensual works of art. But I'll bet the only Japanese art you've seen in museums depicts geishas, landscapes, and flowers. Find a book of Japanese erotica, preferably one containing "spring drawings," their most explicit sexual art.

This variation tweaks the rear-entry position slightly, yet once again creates new sensations for both partners.

1. She gets down on all fours on the bed (or floor) and lowers her head and chest to the mattress, brining her knees forward to elevate her ass at a steep angle.

2. He stands behind her. Holding her hips, he leans forward over her body so that his head is touching (or nearly so, depending on his height) her upper back.

3. He enters her from this position, stimulating her G-spot and clitoris as he thrusts. The pose limits his movement, making intercourse last longer.

....

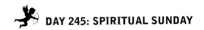 **DAY 245: SPIRITUAL SUNDAY**

Discovering Your Yin and Yang Energies

In Taoist philosophy, everything has an equal and opposite reaction. (Remind you of physics?) Yin and yang are the opposing Tao forces. Yin is passive, negative, and yet nourishing. Yang is the dominant, aggressive, and consuming force. Men were thought to have more yang than yin, and women more yin than yang, with each gender possessing some of the attributes of both. Sex, it was thought, helped a man and a woman keep their yin and yang balanced.

In more recent times, some men have searched for their inner femininity. Usually they were the men who were already in touch with it. Today we question whether the alpha woman can be satisfied by the beta man.

You've been exploring your dominant and submissive sides in some of the daily activities in these pages. Today, pick up your sex journals. Write about how you see yourselves and each other in yin and yang terms. Are there areas you've opened up and would like to explore more fully?

What would Lord Yang and Lady Yin like to do in bed that they haven't done yet?

. . . .

DAY 246: FLIRTATION AND FOREPLAY MONDAY

Whisper the Sexy Compliment

When was the last time you paid your lover a *sexy* compliment? Yes, you say he's handsome and she's beautiful. But how generic is that?

Whisper something good and sexy this morning before you part or tonight before you go to sleep. If you are separated by business, whisper it over the phone. (Please. No text messages.) Make it personal.

Some for inspiration:

- "Your balls smell like musk and spice—and the scent makes me crazy."

- "I love the way your clitoris gets hard and thrusts out when you are turned on."

- "Your cock is perfectly straight and beautiful."

- "I dream about your pussy flexing around my cock."

....

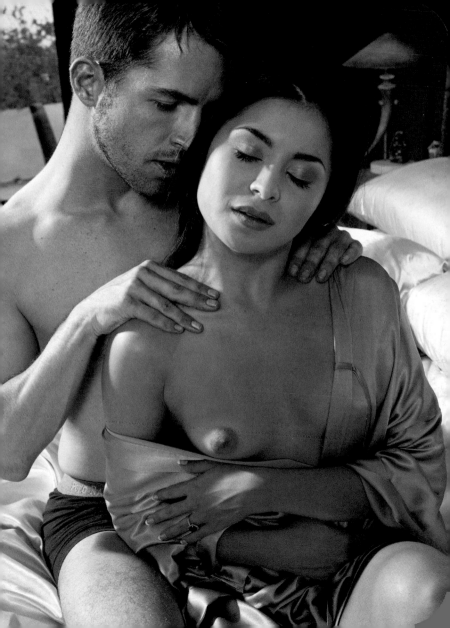

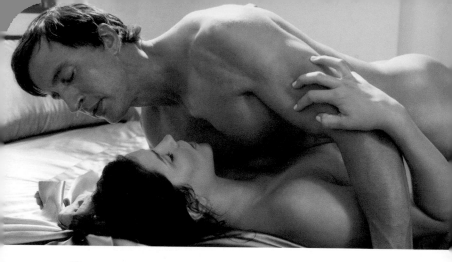

🕐 DAY 247: QUICKIE TUESDAY

The Edge Quickie

Many couples feel like they have been living on the edge these past few years—the thin edge of the time-and-money wedge, so carefully calculated. They balance precariously, hoping their numbers add up. This edge-of-the-bed quickie turns survival energy into sexual energy.

She lies back on the bed, her hips at the edge. He stands in front of her, between her legs.

She raises her legs, placing her ankles on his shoulders. (Put a pillow under the small of her back, if needed.)

Hands under her buttocks (which also helps raise her position to clitoral advantage), he thrusts. Her hands are free to stroke her clit.

. . . .

His Heart in Her Mouth

When you hold a man's cock in your mouth, you are holding his very heart and soul at that moment. Find his heartbeat. Listen to it. That is *your* man.

He sits or stands. You kneel in front of him.

Take his hands in yours. Put your lips on the wrist of one hand and hold it there until you feel his pulse in your lips.

Grasp the shaft of his penis in one hand. Press your lips against it.

As you lick, tongue, and suck his cock in a combination of his favorite moves, keep one hand on his heart. Let the beat guide the pace of your moves.

If you lost track of his heartbeat for a moment, hold his penis in your mouth until you feel it again. Breathe in time with his heartbeat.

Play his cock to that beat as if you were a jazz musician jamming.

You will experience his ejaculation as more satisfying than usual now.

....

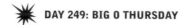 **DAY 249: BIG O THURSDAY**

The Sensuous Orgasm

You created a circle of fire and burned your orgasm through it. With some adjustments to your breathing technique, you can turn your orgasm into a warm sensual experience—like coming in a scented pool filled with floating gardenias. Once you become adept at channeling the sexual power of breathing, you will keep finding ways to create new orgasm experiences. Experiment!

Take your time in building arousal so that you are both intensely aroused by the time you reach orgasm.

As soon as you feel orgasm begin, take a sharp breath in and hold it.

Exhale slowly as your orgasm stretches out.

Grunting on the exhalation also helps some people create a more sensual orgasm, with a slightly longer series of contractions.

....

 DAY 250: GET-YOUR-FREAK-ON FRIDAY

Role-Playing: She's the Boss

She is the executive; he is her personal assistant. Or she is the wealthy socialite, and he is her personal trainer. Create your own scenario where she has the money and power and his only means of getting on top is his sexual power.

Foreplay is her telling him what to do and how. Get specific:

- "Take my nipples between your thumb and first fingers and gently squeeze."

- "Lick around the sides of my clit with the *firm* tip of your tongue."

- "Put your hands on my ass and squeeze in time with your sucking."

The more aroused she gets, the more dominant he becomes—for example, ignoring her instructions but giving her something else that she loves.

When she is close to orgasm, she orders him to finish her orally. He refuses. Putting his erection close to her lips, he says, "Suck me."

She fellates him until he is near orgasm. He pulls out of her mouth and takes her vaginally in the man-on-top position.

....

 DAY 251: SEX ED SATURDAY

Advanced Japanese Sex #2:
Lip Service

Ancient Japanese sexuality was more inclusive of oral pleasuring than the other Eastern erotic cultures. While the Kama Sutra relegated fellatio to a footnote (and less than that for cunnilingus), Japanese erotic books contained explicit instructions for oral sex as both foreplay and a sex act destination and included oral erotica as arousal aids. Create your own erotic books celebrating fellatio and cunnilingus.

Look for surviving bits of ancient Japanese erotic poetry and copy your favorite passages into the books.

Cut and paste photos of erotic drawings from the period. (Old art books are your best source. The online source Alibris.com can find almost anything you request.)

Write your own odes to performing oral sex on your lover.

Here are some examples translated from the Japanese to get you started:

If you know how to approach her,

She will mix every night

Her honey with your milk

If the cup is deep,

Plunge your tongue into it several times.

If she sucks the grains of rice

Of which your sake is made,

It will only be the better for it.

....

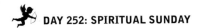 **DAY 252: SPIRITUAL SUNDAY**

Cultivating Electric Energy #1:
The Big Girl's Toy

The male and female currents running through us are electric. Hand him your Hitachi Magic Wand, the big girl's toy, and ask him to give you a full-body electronic massage. Tell him it is an extension of his cock.

Using the Hitachi's original head, he massages your neck, shoulders, and back, then turns you over and runs the vibe up and down your legs and stomach, playing your inner thighs until your insides feel like molten silk.

Switch to the black silicone head with vertical ridges for vulva stimulation on one side and a round ridge for clitoral stimulation on the other. As he skillfully manages the two heads, he kisses your mouth and breasts.

After you've come a few times, he holds the wand between his thighs, in place against you while he plays with your breasts and caresses your hair and face. The motion of his body changes the pattern of the vibrations.

With the Hitachi, you can come over and over with virtually no downtime between orgasms. You know that feeling of helplessness as the desire for orgasm turns into the thing itself and you whimper and give yourself over completely? That feeling goes on . . . and it is the glory of female energy.

Once he has brought this energy up in you, he puts the toy away and enters you, asserting his masculine power all over again.

. . . .

DAY 253: FLIRTATION AND FOREPLAY MONDAY

Make the Sexy Suggestion

A sexy suggestion is the most straightforward—and one of the most effective—forms of mental foreplay. It's so simple, too.

Say, When we have time, I want to...

- "Suck your cock"
- "Lick your clit"
- "Finger your asshole"
- "Put my dick in your mouth"
- "Find that little place on the underside of your penis and flick it 'til you go crazy"
- "Watch you writhe while I play with your clit and fuck you"

....

The Time-Management Quickie #1:
Five Minutes, Five Steps

Set your watches. It is possible to have satisfying (for both partners) sex in five minutes, but you have to know what you're doing and how to do it skillfully. (Longtime lovers have the advantage over strangers in quickies.)

Her foreplay is her responsibility and takes place before the quickie.

1. Grab, kiss, clench, fondle—all at a super-heated, "I'll die if I can't grope you and feel you up" pace. (One minute.)

2. Get into the standing bent-over position (page 159). She puts her hands on a dresser or other piece of furniture for leverage. He nuzzles her neck and lightly slaps her buttocks. (One minute.)

3. He enters her from behind.

4. One or both partners stroke her clitoris as he thrusts, or she wears a sweetheart vibe. (Two and a half minutes.)

5. Orgasm! (Thirty seconds.)

....

The Suburban BJ #1: The Golf Cart

I'm not suggesting you play the course together. That could ruin a good relationship. Head out to drive a few balls. Rent a golf cart. Park it in a quiet spot, some place where lost golf balls go to die.

Sit on his lap and kiss him passionately. When you feel his erection surging inside his pants, get down, take that zipper in your teeth, and set him free.

Hold his penis firmly in one hand. Take the first third into your mouth and work the remaining two-thirds with your hand.

Use the fingers of your other hand to caress his balls and press his perineum.

Make a circular twisting motion up the shaft while you swirl your tongue around the head, flick the corona, and strum the frenulum.

Continue the hand and mouth movements until he is near orgasm. Then suck him to finish.

....

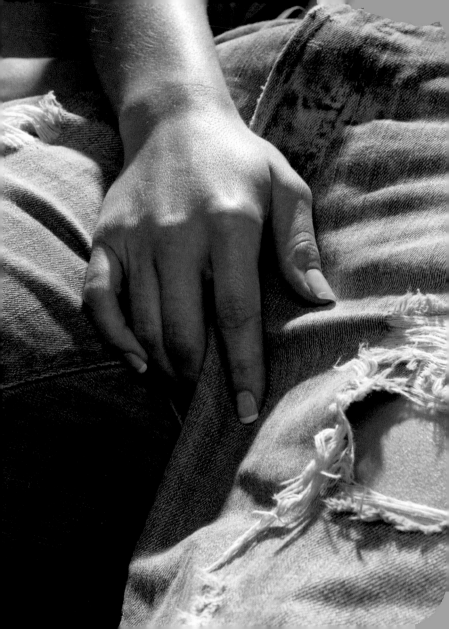

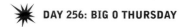 **DAY 256: BIG O THURSDAY**

The AFE Zone Orgasm

The AFE (anterior fornix erotic) zone is one of those spots in the vagina hotly debated by clitoral centrists. You know my position on this: The spots may correlate to parts of the clitoris extending into or behind the vaginal walls, but if women experience them as places *in* the vagina, why argue semantics?

Spongy but not as roughly textured and highly defined as the G-spot, the AFE zone is located closer to the cervix. The Malaysian sexologist Dr. Chua Chee Ann named it based on his study of 193 women. All but eleven reported increased vaginal lubrication and higher arousal when the area was stroked. If this is a sensitive area for you, then see where manual play can take you.

He lies on his back. She mounts him in the female superior position.

As she is leaning back, he inserts two fingers into her vagina and strokes the front wall. He uses light, soft strokes, not the firmer G-spot strokes.

For a variation, she faces his feet in the Reverse Cowgirl position and he uses the same strokes, but coming in from a slightly different angle.

....

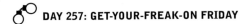 **DAY 257: GET-YOUR-FREAK-ON FRIDAY**

Role-Playing: He's the Boss

Reverse the roles you played last week. He has the power and money. Her only power is sexual (and that is more than good enough).

He orders her to perform some routine tasks, such as straightening his desk and filing. When he tosses a file folder onto the floor and tells her to bend over and pick it up, the game is on.

He makes inappropriate advances for a male authority figure—slapping her ass as she bends over, squeezing her buttocks, brushing his hand across her breasts as she tries to move out of range.

Standing toe-to-toe with her and breathing heavily, he commands her to drop her skirt. Obediently, she does. She isn't wearing panties. He puts his hand between her legs and says, "Open your legs wider."

With his thumb, he roughly massages her clit while his fingers play in her labia. Her cheeks flush and her breathing grows more rapid.

Groaning with desire, he kneels in front of her and licks and sucks her clit.

When she is ready to come, *she* orders him to take off his pants and lie back. She mounts him and rides him to a tremendous climax.

. . . .

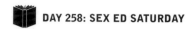

Advanced Japanese Sex #3:
The Supreme Love Gift

Rent *The Teahouse of the August Moon* from Netflix. Read passages from *Memoirs of a Geisha*. Share your erotic oral sex books with one another. Now you are ready to celebrate the supreme gift of your love—the mutual giving of sexual pleasure.

Put a thick rug or several blankets and some pillows on the floor. Dress in your silk kimono.

Sitting cross-legged on the floor, share some warmed sake. Allow your robes to fall open, displaying your genitals. Move closer together, so that your legs can entwine and your hands can reach your lover's genitals.

Imagine that you are lovers in ancient Japan. Create a story together—a story about your passion. Who are you? Royal or servant? What are the obstacles in your path to sharing the supreme love gift?

As you play with one another's genitals and weave your story, be very specific about how you want this celebration to end—taking turns at oral sex? Intercourse—and in what position?

Act out the desired ending.

....

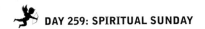 **DAY 259: SPIRITUAL SUNDAY**

Face-to-Face Position #2:
Full Flat Female Superior

The intense face-to-face positions satisfy the craving that men as well as women have for intimate contact. However, they are not always the best positions for reaching orgasm, especially for him. Luckily you don't have to stay in one intercourse position. When you are both ready for him to thrust vigorously (or for her to assume that control on top), change positions. You won't lose the feeling of deep connection.

1. He lies on his back, legs comfortably together. She lies down fully flat on top of him, with the head of his penis rubbing against her clit.

2. Eyes open, they kiss and caress as she moves against his penis (without yet inserting it).

3. When she is ready, she inserts his penis and thrusts by sliding herself up and down on the shaft.

4. She keeps riding him this way until she is ready to reach orgasm. Then she sits up and mounts him. Leaning slightly forward, she thrusts vigorously. He clasps her buttocks in both hands and pushes back.

After they both reach orgasm, she lies on top of him again, resting her head on his chest.

. . . .

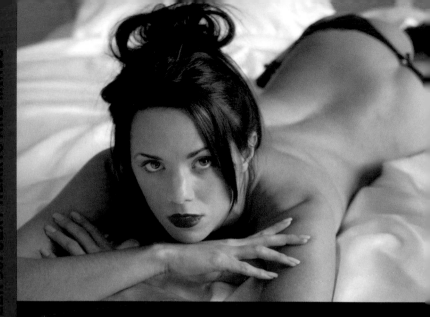

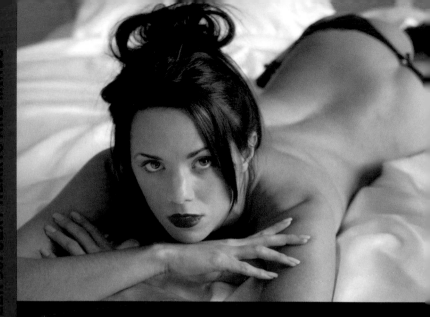 **DAY 260: FLIRTATION AND FOREPLAY MONDAY**

Scalp Massage

You're sitting side by side on the sofa watching TV or in bed reading or working on your laptops. Reach over and caress his (or her) shoulder. Run you fingers up through his hair. Turn toward him and open your arms.

When he moves toward you, guide his head to your breasts. Caress his head.

Using your finger pads, slowly work his scalp in a gentle back-and-forth motion. He may fall asleep in your arms.

....

The Time-Management Quickie #2:
Seven Minutes, Five Steps

You did it in five! Seven is a luxury, right? Again, she is responsible for her own foreplay.

1. The frenzied kissing and groping. (One and a half minutes.)

2. Getting into position. He leans her against the wall. With his help, she either pushes up or pulls off her skirt. No panties (it goes without saying). She wraps one leg around his waist. (One minute.)

3. He clasps one buttock to support her as he enters her, and then thrusts, each stroke deep and slow. (One and a half minutes.)

4. She plays with her clit as he picks up the pace of thrusting, moving more vigorously. (Two and a half minutes.)

5. Orgasm! (Thirty seconds.)

....

The Suburban CJ: The Sunroof

If your car doesn't have an open sunroof, rent or borrow one that does and take her for a drive on a lovely warm day. (A convertible also works as the CJ vehicle.) Insist she wear a sundress, not jeans. Pull off the road in a scenic spot. Open up the sunroof and insist she climb up and put her head out for some fresh air.

Run your hands up and down her legs, caressing her calves and inner thighs. Lick her inner thighs as you pull two finger vibes out of your pocket and put them on, one on each hand.

Lick her labia and follow your tongue with the vibe.

Press your face against her vulva, with the tip of your nose on her clitoris. Keep stroking her labia with the finger vibe as you tickle her clit with your nose.

Purse your lips gently around her clit and circle it with the tip of your tongue. Repeat several times. Add her favorite strokes. Follow every movement of your tongue with a stroke of the finger vibe.

When she is near orgasm, gently suck her clit, repeatedly tapping the tip of it lightly with the tip of your tongue, while two vibrating fingers play with her labia.

....

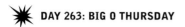 **DAY 263: BIG O THURSDAY**

Orgasmic Providing

Twice I have watched Richard Anton Diaz work his touch magic on a lovely naked model gracing his massage table in a demonstration of Orgasmic Providing. Both were extraordinary events. (I cannot adequately explain the techniques in this space, so go to his website, www.sexyspirits.com, and watch the video presentation.) The man gives orgasms; the women enjoy them.

Anton begins by massaging the woman's entire body before moving, at last, to her vulva. Then, Anton gets into a comfortable position, sitting alongside the model, and spends the next hour taking her to orgasmic peaks, bringing her down into valleys of arousal and back up, using only three fingers.

Depending on how much time is available, your lover can give you a full-body erotic massage, or massage your feet and work his way up your legs to the inner thighs and your vulva. Your lover uses the three middle fingers, placing the outer two above the sides of the clitoral shaft with the others poised to stroke the clitoris. With the outer fingers he exerts slight pressure and moves in very slow up-and-down strokes, picking up the pace when he wants to bring her to orgasm. The middle finger is free to stimulate the shaft.

For further reading, see Bob and Leah Schwartz's, *The One-Hour Orgasm*; Dr. Patricia Taylor's, *Expanded Orgasm*; Margot Anand's, *The Art of Sexual Ecstasy*; and the works of Dr. Victor Baranco.

....

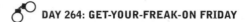

DAY 264: GET-YOUR-FREAK-ON FRIDAY

Fantasy Exploration

Fantasy exploration is a basic tool in the Spice-Up-Your-Sex-Life kit. Yes, fantasy play can be a lot of sexy fun. But tossing off this particular piece of advice—"Explore your fantasies!"—is tantamount to telling someone, "You must be completely honest in your relationship."

Oh, yeah? So honest that you tell him you've had better lovers, or fell for him in spite of his modest endowment, or cheated on her once and wish you hadn't, or fantasize doing it with her best friend?

The Two Big Misconceptions about Fantasies

1. Most people who fantasize SM encounters, group sex, extramarital affairs with their husband's brother, and other common fantasies do *not* want to act them out.

   And fantasizing such things does *not* mean there is something wrong with your relationship.

2. Sex fantasies are powerful arousal tools, but "sharing" indiscriminately kills the arousal.

Here's how to explore your fantasies today: Don't feel guilty about having fantasies. Use them to enrich a masturbation experience, help her "start on warm" before partner sex, and, even during sex, pull out of an arousal slump. A man or woman with a vivid erotic fantasy life most likely also has a hot real sex life.

....

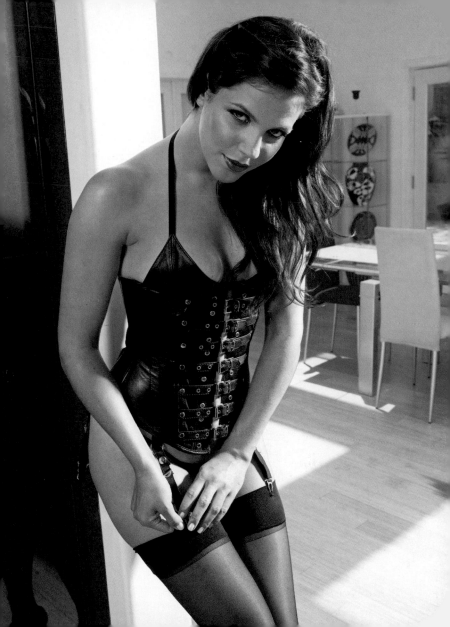

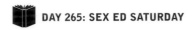

Lady Libido—and the Fire Below

How many millions of women have been told they have a "low libido" (or been labeled "dysfunctional") because they don't feel desire for their partners? A study conducted by Rosemary Basson of the University of British Columbia reports that, in women, desire comes after sex, not before. Once the sex is over, she is finally aroused and feels desire.

"Women often begin sexual experiences feeling sexually neutral," she says. They have sex to please their lover, feel "intimate," short-circuit an argument, make up after a fight, or get what they want or reward the guy for having given it. In Basson's view of female desire, long and sensual lovemaking works best for women because they are slow to arouse. But sometimes there is no time for anything but quickies, and women need to know how to make them work.

Your sex ed assignment today is to create your own Claiming Pleasure Manifesto. For example:

- Don't wait to feel desire simmering way below the surface.

- Jump-start that desire/arousal process by masturbating, particularly with a vibrator as part of foreplay.

- Continue the direct clitoral stimulation during thrusting. Still not satisfied? Ask for oral or manual stimulation to get you there.

Don't silently suffer with your slow-burning Lady Libido. Light a fire under her.

....

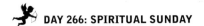 **DAY 266: SPIRITUAL SUNDAY**

Cultivating Electric Energy #2:
The Big We

According to myth, the Greek god Zeus had a three-hundred-year honeymoon with his wife, Hera. His orgasms created the world. Your orgasms can energize your bodies and make you more creative, too.

The new We-Vibe is the first and only internal vibrator designed to be worn during intercourse.

1. She lies back on the bed, legs open wide. He kneels between her legs.

2. Using broad strokes of his tongue, he laps her labia before settling into the familiar rhythm of cunnilingus. He alternates her favorite moves, such as gentle sucking with the fast, teasing flick of the tip of his tongue across the tip of her clit.

3. When she is highly aroused, he inserts the We-Vibe, the cup at one end of the C-shaped vibe over her clit, the other one inside her vagina, surrounding the G-spot.

4. If he is not in a hurry, he can lick and suck her inner thighs while she rocks to orgasm on the We.

5. Finally, he enters her, with the We-Vibe still in place. He will benefit from the vibrations as he thrusts. (The manufacturer promises that the vibe's "slender profile leaves room for penetration." If his cock is large, however, you may have to remove the We.)

. . . .

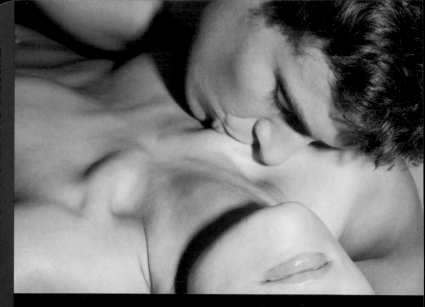

DAY 267: FLIRTATION AND FOREPLAY MONDAY

The Neck Blow

The Kama Sutra encourages men to kiss a woman's neck and to blow on it, especially on a hot day.

Come up behind her. If she has long hair, lift it up, twist it around your fingers, and blow on her exposed neck.

She has short hair?

Come up behind her, and put one arm around her waist and the other hand in her hair. As you run your fingers through her tresses—pulling a little if she likes that—blow on her neck.

....

The Time-Management Quickie #3:
Ten Minutes, Five Steps

A ten-minute quickie is almost a luxury. She may want to stop her private foreplay a little sooner than she did preceding the five- and seven-minute quickies (pages 307 and 315).

1. Ravish one another like lovers who have been separated for weeks. Keep your hands moving purposefully on one another's bodies as you kiss passionately. (Two minutes.)

2. Get into position, with him seated in a chair and her on his lap, her back against his chest. Before entering her, he strokes her clitoris. She teases her nipples and reaches her head back over her shoulder to grab little sucking nibbles at his lips. (Two minutes.)

3. He lifts her up and guides her down onto his erect penis. She plays with her clit while he thrusts slowly. She can lean forward or backward against him to change the coital dynamics. When she wants to increase the pace of intercourse, she uses her legs or arms as leverage. (Three minutes.)

4. She energetically rides him as he thrusts vigorously. (Two and a half minutes.)

5. Orgasm! (Thirty seconds.)

....

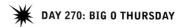 **DAY 269: ORAL WEDNESDAY**

The Bend-Over BJ

One of my favorite SexyPrime male readers (and email correspondents) sent this sex tip, which really works. And it's one of the most popular sex tips on the blog.

He sits on a straight-backed chair. (An overstuffed chair won't work.)
He spreads his legs open. She kneels on a pillow and starts sucking away
with a hand on the nut sack and prostate. Oh, what a feeling, because
you can bend over, reach down, and grab her ass while she's doing this.
You can last a while sitting down; it depends how much you pump her
mouth. Last time, she let me cum inside her mouth, then popped her lus-
cious lips right under the head, which makes for an incredible sensation.
This kept me hard afterward for some doggie-style . . . yum.

. . . .

DAY 270: BIG O THURSDAY

Visualizing Arousal

The first step in the Orgasm Loop—the no-fail technique I created for reaching orgasm—is to visualize arousal. If women can "see" arousal, they can't deny it. Could a man deny his erection? Numerous studies have shown, however, that women routinely deny arousal. Hooked up to sensors, watching erotic videos, many say, "I'm not aroused by that porn!" though their heart and breathing rates are elevated and their vaginas are lubricating. In denying arousal, they short-circuit their own orgasms.

Further complicating the issue, we get confused between desire and arousal. For decades, sex researchers and therapists accepted the model of sexual response developed in the 1960s by Dr. William Masters and Dr. Virginia Johnson: Desire precedes arousal. New studies contradict that. Neurobiologists report that women's brains are blazing with arousal before they even experience desire for a sexual encounter.

1. Close your eyes, clear your mind of distractions, and visualize your own arousal.

2. Create your arousal image. Some women, for instance, might visualize their genitalia—lips sweating and moisture forming, the color changing to deeper pink. Other women might visualize a flower, perhaps an orchid. Some women might see arousal as a color, perhaps pink, red, or saffron yellow, the color of Saraswati, the Hindu goddess of knowledge and the arts who embodies the wisdom of Devi, mother goddess in Hindu mythology.

3. Focus on your arousal image every time you use the Orgasm Loop. It is the mental equivalent of an erotic mantra.

. . . .

DAY 271: GET-YOUR-FREAK-ON FRIDAY

Thinking Off

Can you think yourself to a no-hands orgasm? Maybe.

The most interesting sex research in the nation—probably the world—is being conducted in a Rutger's lab by a brilliant team under the direction

(continued on next page)

of Dr. Barry Komisaruk. Their findings should (and probably won't) put to rest the clitoral versus vaginal orgasm debate. Women are so complex that some of us can come without direct stimulation to either area. Do the highly orgasmic test subjects, however, flex their PC (pubococcygeal) muscle while thinking off? I would bet at least some do.

The Orgasm Loop has four parts: mental arousal image (see page 324); Tantric breathing; PC flexing; and energy transfer, as done in martial arts. Any woman can learn the Loop, but she likely won't get it together on the first try. It's like riding a bike. Give it a week.

Try the short version to see whether you have the potential for thinking off:

1. Use the arousal focus technique on page 324.

2. Add fire breathing on page 210.

3. Flex your PC muscle in time with your breathing, tightening on the inhalation, relaxing on the exhalation.

Flexing a well-toned PC can trigger, intensify, or sustain orgasm in a highly aroused woman. I have been able to "think off" on occasion, usually when I am in the throes of new passion. PC flexing is part of the process for me. It might be "no hands" but it isn't "no physical stimulation."

....

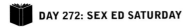

The Art of Sex

Artists have depicted sexuality since the first caveman or woman drew stick figures on the walls. Sadly, if you are an American citizen, you will be able to find very little erotic art in museums. But, you can find beautifully erotic art books filled with photos of paintings, drawings, and sculptures that will touch your soul and stir your mind, as well as your genitals.

In *The Art of Arousal*, a collection of erotic counters by famous artists, Dr. Ruth Westheimer celebrates a range of pieces, including Titian's dreamy romantic reclining nudes, Paul Cezanne's *Afternoon in Naples*, Aubrey Beardsley's witty erotic drawings, George Grosz's pigs dressed as men cavorting with naked women, Toulouse-Lautrec's French whores, Shunga art, and so much more.

Dr. Ruth writes, "Sex has been one of the principal concerns of art in all cultures, and the finest artists of all times have made the human body the instrument of beauty and feeling."

Look at erotic art today. What does it say to you? How does it inspire you? Share your opinions about the art you see, and maybe learn something new about each other.

....

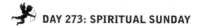 **DAY 273: SPIRITUAL SUNDAY**

Building the Long Desire:
Attraction Plus Obstacles

In *The Erotic Mind,* Jack Morin posited this simple formula for hot sex:

ATTRACTION + OBSTACLES = EXCITEMENT

Romantic comedies are created on the concept. Once the attracted couple overcome the obstacles and get together, the movie ends before the excitement cools. Sometimes it seems that modern Western society must be the most (foolishly) romantic of all time. But the ancient Egyptians were as sentimental and romantic about love as we are.

Their word for love, loosely translated, means "a long desire." Their love poems—and Shakespeare's plays, for that matter—are filled with separations and calamities that keep lovers apart. These sometimes tragic lovers exist in the state of *ragavat,* the passionate love of the Kama Sutra, born of intense physical attraction.

What is the message for a couple trying to balance love and life and hoping to create and sustain a long desire? Great sex—the sustaining of *ragavat,* or the long desire—requires balancing intimacy and separateness. In America, we overemphasize intimacy at the expense of separateness.

"Let there be spaces in your togetherness," Khalil Gibran said in *The Prophet.* Space is an aphrodisiac. Give each other some space today.

....

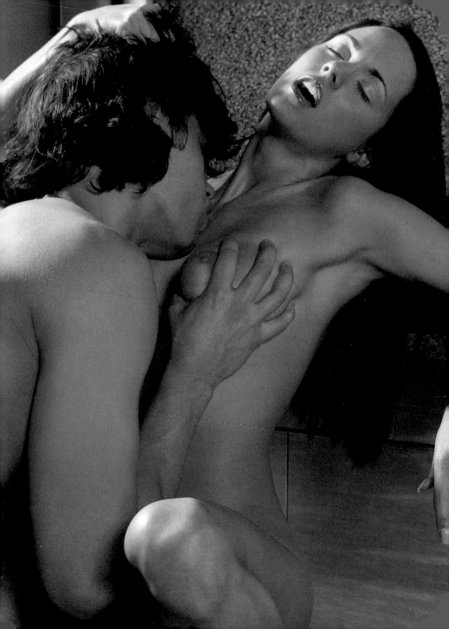

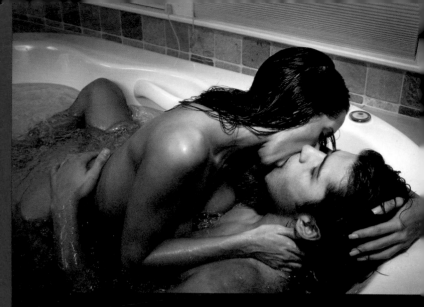

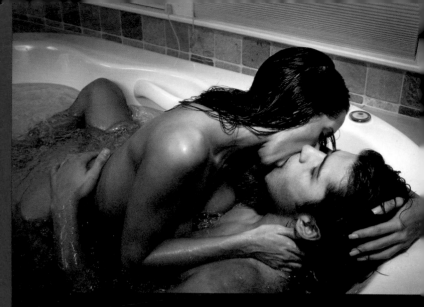 **DAY 274: FLIRTATION AND FOREPLAY MONDAY**

The Wet Look

You know the power of looking at your lover from across the room and moistening your lips. Wet is sexy.

Don't put up your umbrella in a fine mist. Meet your man for dinner with the mist in your hair and the "dew" on your cheeks.

No rain?

An exotic dancer I interviewed a few years back told me she sprays a light mist of scented oil on her throat and chest before a date. In the candlelight, her cleavage gleams softly.

....

The Bend-Over Cross Quickie

I created this variation on a classic position for *The New Tantra: Simple and Sexy*. The photograph of this pose is one of my favorite shots in that beautiful little book. I was on set for the shoot, and what a privilege that was.

The bend-over is a classic quickie intercourse position. She stands with feet apart. If she's athletic, she bends forward and places her hands on the floor. He enters from behind. Most of us do the bend-over in a more comfortable position, such as standing but leaning forward with hands or forearms supported by a bed, table, chair, or other hard surface while he enters from behind. Here's my adaptation:

Preferably wearing stilettos because they look so hot, assume your favorite bend-over position, but cross your ankles after he enters you. The fit feels tighter and more exciting for him and stimulates your G-spot or clitoris indirectly. Flex your PC muscle in time with his thrusting to intensify the sensations.

. . . .

DAY 276: ORAL WEDNESDAY

The Cunnilingus Quickie

Want to turn cunnilingus into the ultimate oral quickie—or at least a Cunnilingus Quickie? Alternate mouth stimulation with the clever use of a little bullet vibe. Here's the ultra-simple technique:

1. Cover her clitoris with her labia lips to protect the ultrasensitive clit from vibe stimulation that might otherwise feel too intense, even painful. You can also leave her silk panties in place for this part.

2. If the vibe has two speeds, start on low and move to high if her body language indicates she wants that.

3. When she's close to orgasm, turn off the vibe and put that mouth back on the job.

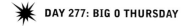

DAY 277: BIG O THURSDAY

The Sleep Orgasm

Sleep orgasms are not for men only. Women have our own version of the "wet dream." Dr. Alfred Kinsey reported back in 1953 that 40 percent of women would experience at least one sleep orgasm before they turned forty. A casual comment, a line from an email, or an image—maybe graphic, maybe not—all drift into the sex brain, where they get caught up in pulsating waves of desire. Before you realize what's happening, your restless tossing and turning has rubbed your clit the right way.

There is no way to make sleep orgasms happen, but you can be open to the possibility: encourage sexy thoughts or play with your clit before falling asleep.

Here's a story from my blog SexyPrime:

It happened to me again a few nights ago. I woke to an orgasm and the fantasy of an encounter with a man dominating me in bed. He was familiar, yet not. A woman is never so submissive as when she offers her ass to a man, and that vulnerable state is even more thrilling if he is neither stranger nor lover. Thrusting his dick rhythmically into my anus, he occasionally slapped each cheek. The sound of smacks on sweating flesh echoed in my head. I closed my eyes and felt his hot breath behind me. Here's the thing about anal sex: if you're into it at the moment, it hurts so good. (The porn films never get it right.) And I was into it. I played with my clit as he rammed in and out of me, and I came.

He withdrew, turned me over, pulled off the condom, and tossed it. I thought he was going to fuck me, but he picked up his belt from the floor and ordered, "Spread your legs open wide."

Legs widespread, hand in pussy, I moved my hips up toward him as he lightly hit my inner thighs with his belt. I was straining to come, gasping and pulling deep inside for an orgasm that made me work for it. He put down the belt, entered me, fucked me hard and fast, and I came and came. His face close to mine still wasn't quite clear. I fell back asleep with my hand in my pussy. In the morning, I thought: I need to call him.

....

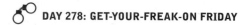 **DAY 278: GET-YOUR-FREAK-ON FRIDAY**

Fantasy Scripts

The Three Golden Rules of Fantasies

1. A fantasy is often not a wish or desire and rarely provides a road map to a potential real sex encounter, but it is a healthy way of exploring your sexual taboos, such as a spontaneous sexual encounter with a stranger, multiple partners, "taboo" practices such as BDSM and exhibitionism, or "forced sex."

2. Once you share a fantasy, you may rob it of its power to arouse. It's not your private little secret anymore.

3. We are all aroused by things we don't want to do, and there's nothing wrong with that. Sharing fantasies can be thrilling, but share those fantasies carefully and act them out with even greater care.

- Take turns selecting or writing erotic fantasies to read as part of foreplay.

- Read a fantasy while your partner masturbates.

- Use the fantasies as phone sex scripts when you're not together.

- If you want to act out one of your scenarios, develop the details together as if you were erotic screenwriters. Remember: Much of fantasy play is theater. You pretend your lover is a stranger and pick him up in a bar, then give him a blow job in the car. When in doubt, dial it down.

....

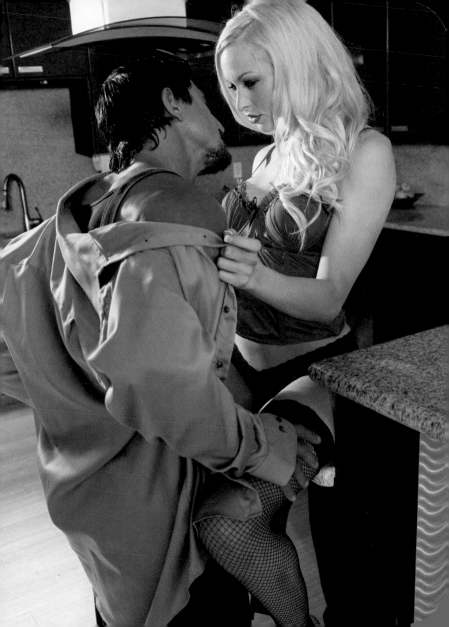

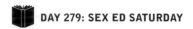

Handling His Desire Curve

Men have desire curves, too. Their sexual performance is even more affected than hers by a range of factors, including being overweight, a sedentary lifestyle, prescription and recreational drugs, and alcohol. Ironically, his fall from New Relationship Euphoria (NREU) sometimes leads him to use recreational drugs and alcohol to increase desire. (Big mistake.)

NREU is a chemical high (see page 177). The first neurotransmitter chemical firing off in your brain when you are strongly attracted to someone new is phenylethylamine (PEA), a natural form of amphetamine, influencing sexual arousal. Norepinephrine, a second euphoria-inducing chemical, kicks in and elevates blood pressure. PEA releases dopamine, the body's "feel good" neurochemical, stimulating the production of oxytocin, dubbed the "cuddle chemical" because it encourages bonding and attachment. This powerful cocktail of brain chemicals creates a state of euphoria, intensified by intercourse and orgasm.

What can you do when the high trends down?

1. Accept that you cannot sustain a NREU high throughout the decades. You can, however, create peaks in your valleys, a pattern of undulating waves of desire.

2. Don't make reckless choices. Standing up for monogamy is not my job. You make your own decisions—but make them from knowledge of sex science, not fear, such as the fear of losing your sexual potency or being stuck in a marriage without passion.

3. Don't expect her to make all the effort at reviving your sex life when it slumps. Take an active role.

4. Break sexual habits. Habituation is deadly in a sexual relationship. You have to shake it up. Learn some new tricks.

5. Do what scares you a little, which might mean taking more emotional risks with your woman, opening up, and sharing your fears and desires.

. . . .

 DAY 280: SPIRITUAL SUNDAY

Sex Rituals

Sex is part ritual. Like religion, sex incorporates habitual elements that give it special meaning. Repeating some of these habits contribute to the feeling that sex has become routine.

Cultivate the ritual aspects of lovemaking without falling into a rut. Some suggestions:

- Candles
- Flowers
- Special clothing

- Incense
- Music

Physical gestures, such as holding out a hand to initiate the walk into the bedroom, taking her face in his hands, or putting her hand on his thigh.

But doing it the same way every time isn't sex ritual—it's sex rut.

. . . .

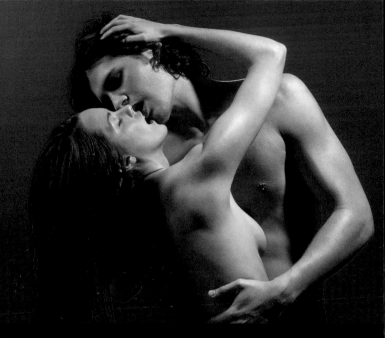

DAY 281: FLIRTATION AND FOREPLAY MONDAY

The Lip Pulse Kiss

Can a quick kiss make your lover's lips pulse? Yes. And you don't have to bite him to make that happen.

Hold your mouth to his wrist until you feel his pulse in your lips.

Quickly press your lips firmly against his.

Suck each lip individually and press your closed lips firmly against his again. You have brought his pulse into his lips—and yours.

....

The Hands-On Quickie

You may have noticed that I've said many times, "She probably needs direct clitoral stimulation to reach orgasm," so:

- She touches herself or he does while thrusting.

- She (or he) uses a small vibe on her clit during thrusting.

- You tweak positions, including the use of pillows, to get more indirect clitoral stimulation during thrusting.

In the Hands-on Quickie, he leaves the clit play to her, but he uses his hands in creative ways all over her body and with intensity.

1. She lies on her back with her ass close to the edge of the bed. He stands in between her legs.

2. He presses his forearm against her vulva while caressing her thighs with the other hand.

3. While she plays with her clit, he runs his hands up and down her arms and legs. Caressing her buttocks, he inserts his penis.

4. He continues caressing her body as he thrusts, and she takes care of her clit.

. . . .

The Folded Deck Chair, Hers

Here's another tip from a male SexyPrime reader—and a great one! I don't know why women readers don't send in more tips. (Any thoughts on that?)

The two strokes that I employ when I want my wife to climb the walls are backdoor penetration (analingus, finger play), which I can do only when she's feeling up to it, and my personal favorite, the Folded Deck Chair.

She lies on her back with her legs open. He kneels between them.

She lifts her legs to rest comfortably on his shoulders, giving him full access to her vulva, clitoris, and G-spot for manual stimulation.

He begins with broad tongue strokes of her labia, starting from the bottom and up to her clitoris, then adds a hand or vibe for G-spot stimulation.

He switches to a finger vibe and stimulates her perineum and labia as he performs her favorite clitoral moves.

After bringing her to one orgasm, they have intercourse in this position, which allows for deeper penetration and is more enjoyable for when she is really "open" following oral orgasm.

....

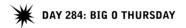 **DAY 284: BIG O THURSDAY**

Her Intercourse Orgasm

Women still want to know: "How can I come during intercourse?"

1. Use manual stimulation during intercourse, in any position.

With his hand or yours or a vibe, stroke. That's the short answer. If you are shy, try this technique:

The Flying V

Many women find this simple technique more effective for inducing orgasm than directly stroking or circling the clitoris, especially during intercourse, when the space available between bodies does limit the options a bit. The bonus? It looks like you are playing with him because you are holding his penis in the wide part of the V.

- Insert two fingers of one hand between your bodies. Form an upside-down V shape, with your fingers straddling your clitoris and his penis. Press the V in time with his thrusting.

- Or take his fingers and place them in the V shape on the sides of your clitoris. Grind against his fingers as he thrusts.

2. Forego "ladies first."

If he typically brings you to orgasm via cunnilingus, then has his O during intercourse, stop him before things proceed to their inevitable conclusions. This increases the likelihood that you will come during intercourse.

3. Do your own foreplay.

Masturbate to the point where orgasm is imminent before grabbing that man, throwing him down on the bed, and mounting him.

4. Tweak the basics.

There are so many ways you can adapt intercourse positions to get more of the clitoral and G-spot friction you need. Add pillows. Shift the angle and depth of penetration by rearranging your bodies.

5. Learn the Orgasm Loop.

I created it, and it works! If orgasm is problematic for you, then buy *The Orgasm Loop*, a complete course in orgasm.

············

 DAY 285: GET-YOUR-FREAK-ON FRIDAY

The SM Fantasy

As I said a few weeks ago, most women (and men) do not want to act out their SM fantasies as aggressively as they imagine them. Some do, and that's fine, too, as long as everyone is on the same page. You may find that reading SM stories is nice foreplay for down-and-dirty sex that leaves you sore in a good way, but not marked.

Here is one from a SexyPrime reader, a man in his early forties:

It started with a mutual admiration for the literary qualities and arousal power of The Story of O and some herbal relaxation of inhibitions. She liked to be spanked. She asked me to pull her hair while we were fucking. No, harder, really hard! We went shopping in a hardware store and she tried on dog collars in the aisle. We ended up deciding that leather beat metal cuffs for us. She asked me to slap her face while we were going at it, not hard, not to leave marks, just enough to get her off even more than she was already getting off. When she asked me to use my

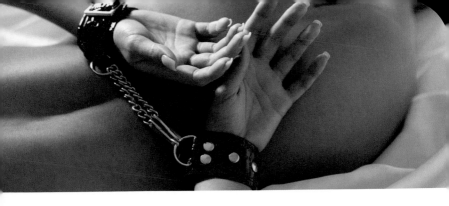

belt, she did want marks on her backside and she wanted me to fuck her from behind while her ass was still burning from the stripes—and she said she loved it that way because it made her feel like I was using her and that got her off even more.

She liked to please. She liked not having to decide. She liked to suck cock. She liked to take it deep and she liked it when I took control. I hadn't really ever seen myself as the Master type (and still don't, really, although I know that I can do it and I know that it can really arouse me), but I do like the woman I'm with to get plenty of whatever gets her off, and she got off on submission, some pain, and surrender of control, and so that's what I gave her. It turned out that it got me off really well, too, but I think that was as much about seeing her powerful response and feeling a sense of power at being able to take it further and further the more she showed what she wanted. She liked being played with, feeling a little used, obeying orders, and getting off thereby. I liked fucking her while she was getting off, and it was a marvelous mutual feedback arousal and release system while it lasted.

....

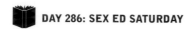

Handling Her Desire Curve

Women are hit harder by their fall from the top of the Desire Curve (pages 177 and 336) than men are. Why? Three reasons:

1. New Relationship Euphoria (NREU) gives women the bigger kick because sex, especially if it includes intercourse and orgasm, adds *large* amounts of the attachment chemical oxytocin to the rush of neurochemicals already bathing her fevered brain. Women are also more affected by oxytocin than men are because it works in concert with estrogen and is somewhat subdued by testosterone. Intercourse produces more oxytocin in women than cunnilingus and other sex acts do.

2. Women confuse desire and arousal and ignore the signs of their own arousal. The myths surrounding "Lady Libido" (page 320) only confuse the situation more.

3. Culturally, women still link love and sex more than men do. The flip side of romanticizing lust and confusing it with love is confusing a fall from NREU with falling out of love.

When you understand the Desire Curve, you can relax and be grateful for the natural hormonal cycles that make you crave again. And remember: Nothing tricks the lust brain like a change of sexual habit. This book is all about beating the Desire Curve.

············

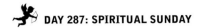 **DAY 287: SPIRITUAL SUNDAY**

The Long Embrace #1: Karezza

An Italian word that means "caress," *karezza* was adapted in the 1880s from Tantric and Taoist teachings by a minister, a founding member of the Oneida Community, and an American physician, Alice Bunker Stockham. A woman ahead of her time, Stockham had her patients prepare for karezza by reading uplifting writings, such as the poems of Elizabeth Barrett Browning and the philosophy of Ralph Waldo Emerson. And she thought lovers should hold the intercourse position for an hour. "Discuss the writings you have read during this period of tranquil sexual union," she lectured. (One may assume she was a virgin.)

Karezza prolongs intercourse and encourages extended orgasm. For the jaded sophisticate, it is a new way to make love. For the harried modern couple, it's a Sunday or vacation erotic exploration.

Dramatically limit his genital movement in either the female superior or the side-by-side position. He does not move inside her unless he becomes flaccid, and then he executes only a few shallow thrusts to revive his erection. But he strokes her breasts and clitoris.

She takes charge of movement, including thrusting her hips against him or contracting her PC muscle around his penis. No matter how excited she gets, he thrusts only enough to sustain his erection.

He holds their lovemaking embrace until she has achieved at least one and preferably more orgasms.

....

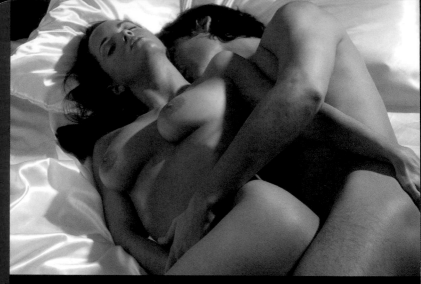

 DAY 288: FLIRTATION AND FOREPLAY MONDAY

The Pelvic Thrust Hug

We hug family members and friends from the waist up, with our pelvises pushed back so as not to touch "inappropriately." In a society where even business associates sometimes hug, people are so accustomed to the pelvis-pulled-back hug that they give the same kind of casual hug to their lovers.

Put your pelvis into your hug today—when there is no opportunity for "sex."

Put your arms around your man (or woman) and hug with your full body, thrusting your pelvis into his.

. . . .

The Cowgirl Vibrating Quickie

This cowgirl is ready to rope and ride her man. Already aroused by vibe play, she's dressed for the part before he comes into the room. Wearing a cowgirl hat (or a reasonable facsimile), boots, and a strap-on vibe, she lassoes him (with a scarf or fabric belt) and orders him to take off his pants.

With one hand, she pushes him backward down on to the bed.

Without removing her boots, she mounts him and rides to climax by moving in an oval track rather than up and down. Imagine you are circumscribing an oval with your body, with the downstroke at one end of the oval and the upstroke at the other. Lean slightly forward as you push down on his penis, stimulating your clitoris. Pull up and move slightly backward on the upstroke, stimulating your G-spot.

. . . .

The No-Touch (His Penis) BJ

A good BJ is usually part hand job. The key to this no-hands BJ is *super heat*. You are both *so* aroused that the sexual energy is reverberating back and forth between you. At that point, his cock doesn't need hand support.

1. She kneels in front of him. He is either standing or sitting on a chair or at the edge of the bed.

2. Without using his hands, he guides his cock toward her open mouth. She wraps her lips around it and, in the welcoming move, slides those lips as far down the shaft as she comfortably can.

3. Sliding her mouth up and down his shaft, she makes eye contact with him and lets her moans sigh against his cock. She swirls her tongue around the head on the upstroke. (She can put her hands on his thighs but not his buttocks, because that would influence his thrusting.)

4. Alternate the sliding/swirling with firm "nibbling" kisses up and down his shaft, strumming the frenulum and flicking/sucking the corona.

5. Suck the head. Imagine you are pulling the ejaculate up his shaft.

6. When he is ready to come, she positions herself so she can take him as deeply as possible.

....

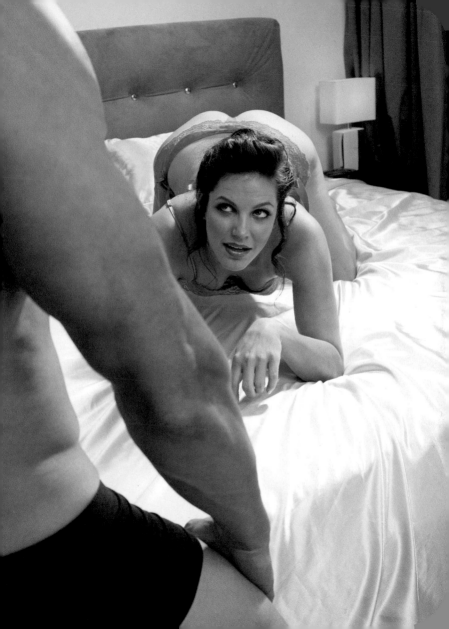

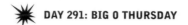 **DAY 291: BIG O THURSDAY**

Is It "Sex" If You Don't Orgasm?

Research conducted in a new study from the Kinsey Institute at Indiana University found that there is "no universal consensus on which behaviors constituted having 'had sex.'"

In the study, 486 Indiana residents were asked in phone interviews, "Would you say you 'had sex' with someone if the most intimate behavior you engaged in was . . ." followed by fourteen behaviorally specific activities. Some results:

- 95 percent of respondents said that penile-vaginal intercourse counted as having "had sex"

- 89 percent said penile-vaginal intercourse was sex only if the male had ejaculated

- 30 percent didn't consider oral sex "sex"

- 20 percent didn't count anal sex as "sex"

But, they did not ask, "Is it sex if the woman doesn't orgasm?"

What do you think? Weeks ago, I asked you to redefine sex. What does your new definition look like? Does it include her orgasm—or not?

....

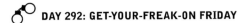 **DAY 292: GET-YOUR-FREAK-ON FRIDAY**

The "Overtaken" Fantasy

Women do fantasize about being "overtaken," but not in a brutal way. The classic "rape fantasy" is the erotic extension of the fairy tale myths of our girlhood. Sleeping Beauty. Cinderella. Snow White. The fair maidens do not choose; they are chosen. They do not act; they are acted upon. The prince awakens them. If you doubt the lingering power of that myth, ponder this: Why else would so many women be reluctant to touch themselves during intercourse, ensuring their own orgasms? The deep desire to be transported on the penis alone is the sexual awakening myth.

In our big girl fantasies, he wants us so badly that he rips off our panties. (Read any romance novels lately?) But, he is the prince, always the prince, who satisfies us completely, and not that icky troll living under the bridge.

According to an article in *The Journal of Sex Research*, between one-third and one-half of women have had the fantasy. The conventional wisdom of therapists holds that it gives women permission to enjoy sexuality. ("The girl can't help it.")

Whatever its roots, the fantasy of romantic ravishment creates conflict in some women and confusion in men. Tell him your fantasies. Talk about what they really mean. He probably doesn't realize how important those princess myths have been in the lives of little girls and women.

Relax and enjoy your fantasy—and know that fantasizing a romanticized takeover does not mean you want to be attacked.

．．．．．．．．．．．．

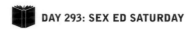

DAY 293: SEX ED SATURDAY

Dance Lessons #1: Pole Dancing

Demi Moore's film *Striptease* was critically panned, but it had a lasting impact on the culture by bringing stripper poles into suburban garages, dens, and bedrooms. Pole-dancing classes are not enough for some women. They must possess the pole.

Pole dancing is performance art, combining dance with gymnastics, and it's a good aerobic workout and strengthens upper body and core muscle groups. Believe it or not, it may also become an Olympic sport.

Watch a video on pole dancing together. Do you both find it arousing? Take a class. They're easy to find. Order a pole if you have the room.

Surprise your man tonight by spinning around the bed pole (or whatever else you can find to support a spin) wearing nothing but stilettos and posing with one leg raised or around the pole, your back arched and head back. A come-get-me look from this position will receive an immediate and enthusiastic response.

············

DAY 294: SPIRITUAL SUNDAY

The Long Embrace #2: Kabazzah

Thousands of years ago in the Middle East, a woman who had mastered the art of "pompoir" (page 145), control of the PC muscle during intercourse, was called a kabazzah, or "one who holds." Kabazzahs were the best prostitutes. Their lifestyle was equivalent to that enjoyed today by the most expensive call girls.

Kabazzah (the technique) has long been a specialty of Asian call girls too, particularly Japanese prostitutes. American soldiers in World War II and Vietnam discovered kabazzah on R&R leaves.

For kabazzah to work, he must be in a relaxed and passive state of mind and body. She must have mastery of her PC muscle through Kegels, which she has practiced for at least a month. The female superior and sitting positions work best for most couples.

1. She stimulates her lover until he is just erect, not highly aroused. Then she inserts his penis.

2. He does not move his penis at all. Never. Not once.

3. She also strives for no pelvic movement, confining movement as much as possible to only her PC muscle.

4. They kiss and caress each other freely.

5. She flexes her PC muscle in varying patterns until, after ten to fifteen minutes, she feels his penis throbbing.

6. She times her contractions to the throbbing of his penis, clenching and releasing in time with him.

7. He will experience a longer, more intense orgasm than normal. After his orgasm, she can flex her PC muscle like crazy and have an orgasm of her own.

....

DAY 295: FLIRTATION AND FOREPLAY MONDAY

Wake Up Your Vagina

These two sexercises will help stimulate the sexual nerve endings in your pelvic region. They are good for any woman of any age. And you look hot doing them.

The Sexy Squat

Stand with feet shoulder-width apart and slowly lower your butt as if you were going to sit in a chair. Squeeze your PC muscle and the muscles in your buttocks as you rise back up. Do several squats three times daily.

The Seat

Sit back on your heels and reach your arms forward. Hold for one minute, then sit up and lean back as far as you can, hands on the floor behind you for support. Hold for one minute. Do several seats three times daily.

....

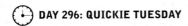

No-Panties-Day Quickie

She announces she's not wearing any panties today. He salivates. And she says, "You plan the quickie—and I'll be ready."

He comes up with an original quickie dependent on location for its appeal, such as in the backseat of the car parked in the garage, some deserted public place, the laundry room, deck, or pool; or a quickie fantasy game to be acted out in their own bedroom; or a quickie with arousal quotient in the execution (the combination of foreplay strokes and intercourse moves).

He texts her the plan, including time and place. If there are arrangements to be made or accessories to be purchased, he handles it.

She is responsible for her own pre-quickie foreplay.

Next time, he announces he's going commando and the quickie planning is up to her.

············

The "Make Him Come" BJ

Some men say that they cannot reach orgasm via oral sex (or come in a woman's mouth). What could be stopping them? They may be reluctant to surrender control, inhibited or worried or angry, or on Viagra. You can overcome *anything* with this BJ. Assert your erotic power.

The key element: Stroke your clit while you are fellating him. Watching your pleasure will add to his excitement and definitely remove his mental roadblock into the pleasure zone.

1. Keeping one hand firmly around the base of his penis (while the other is in your pussy), work the shaft only in upstrokes.

2. Suck his penis by pulling in your cheeks and releasing them. It's not necessary to take in more than the head, corona, and top of the shaft. Suck in time with your upward hand strokes. Let your own panting set the pace for your rhythmic moves.

3. Alternate the sucking with licking the corona, swirling your tongue around the head, and strumming the frenulum, but keep going back to the suck.

4. When you are close to orgasm, tear your hand away from your clit. Take his penis in both hands, fingers laced together. Create a pulsing movement with your hands. Work that movement up his penis. When you get to the head, add a little suck as you pulsate him.

5. If he hasn't come in your mouth yet, repeat the steps. He will.

....

COLES

11/22/2013 16:36
Store# 00704 Term# 003 Trans# 438157

DEFECT

Attach Receipt to Defective Item

RECEIPT NOT VALID FOR STORE RETURNS

DAILY SEX BIBLE $-19.99
9731592334476
Reason: (070) DAMAGED
Orig Str# 00704 Term# 003 Trans# 438066

Holiday refunds accepted until
January 12, 2014. Items brought
back with a gift receipt and in
store-bought condition may be
exchanged for a credit note for the
value of the item on the receipt.

007040030438157 9

Store# 00704 Term# 003 Trans# 438157

Refunds or exchanges may be made within 14 days if item is returned in re-bought condition with a receipt. Items with a gift receipt may be exchanged refunded onto a credit note for the value of the item at the time of purchase. We cannot provide an exchange or refund on magazines or newspapers.

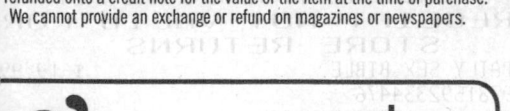
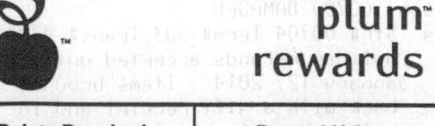

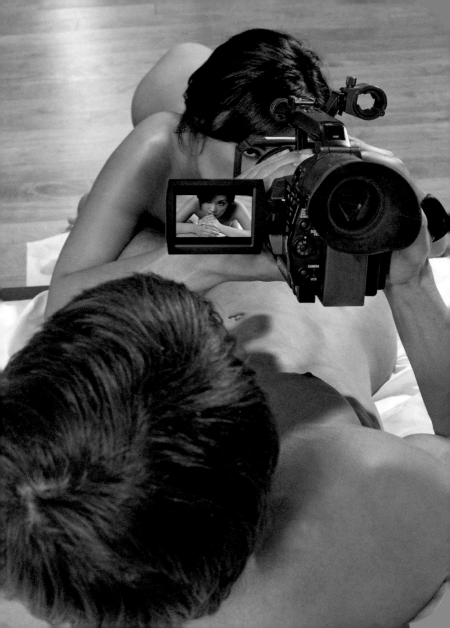

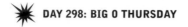 **DAY 298: BIG O THURSDAY**

Four Easy Steps to Multiple Os

You've used the physical techniques for encouraging multiple orgasms during cunnilingus, manual stimulation, and intercourse (page 270). These four simple steps will also make multiple orgasms more likely.

Pre-arousal

Indulge your sensual side on a daily basis—and especially before sex. Ask him to apply body lotion for you, rub you down with rose petals on his finger pads, and shampoo and brush your hair.

Mental Imaging

Imagine pleasure. See yourself in the throes of orgasm. Fantasize sexual encounters.

Vibe Play

Use a vibrator with him in foreplay and alone as pre-foreplay. If you have one or more orgasms in vibe play, you are likely to keep them rolling.

Clitoral Focus

Keep a hand or vibe on your clitoris or nearby during oral stimulation and intercourse. Continue to focus on your clit after an orgasm.

. . . .

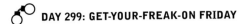

Taking It Out #1: Cuddle Parties

Reid Mihalko, a bicoastal sex educator known as the Cuddle Party Man, may not have invented cuddle parties, but he made them part of the sex culture. An event he held in New York City some years ago captured the attention of the national media, who went with the storyline that "New Yorkers have to pay to cuddle." (Really—we can cuddle for free, but who has the time to invest in wooing a partner?)

Check sex event venues in your area. If you live in an urban area, there may be a cuddle party event near you. If not, throw your own cuddle party. That way, you get to make the rules.

It's not a cuddle party if:

- Clothes are removed.

- Genitals are fondled.

- Sex acts are performed. (Yes, a BJ is a sex act.)

- Couples wander off to be alone.

- Anything other than fully clothed public cuddling occurs.

Some couples may be okay with cuddling others; some may not be. If the party is primarily couples, singles may not feel welcome. Think through the guest list carefully.

. . . .

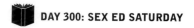 **DAY 300: SEX ED SATURDAY**

Dance Lessons #2: Belly Dancing

Belly dancing has its roots in India, Iran, and Africa, where it grew out of moves that women made to ease the pain of childbirth. (Yes, really.) Napoleon discovered belly dancers when he invaded Egypt in 1798. In Philadelphia, a dancer named Little Egypt stole the show at the 1876 centennial celebration. Today, the Latin pop star Shakira has made the dance her own and singer/dancers including Britney Spears, Jessica Simpson, and Beyoncé incorporate the moves into their routines.

Isn't it time you shook a little hips and belly for your man?

- Watch a video together. Is it arousing for both of you?

- Take a class or learn from instructional DVDs.

- Surprise him with a seductive dance when you have mastered the basics.

- Incorporate some of the moves into sex; for example, work that belly in the female superior position.

....

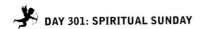

DAY 301: SPIRITUAL SUNDAY

The Tantra Yab-Yum Position

The Yab-Yum is a position for leisurely lovemaking. Light candles, burn incense, arrange fresh flowers in a vase on the bedside table, and play soft music. Lie in each other's arms. Stroke and caress and fondle each part of the other's body, except the genitals. Devote as much time to this luxurious state of foreplay as necessary to reach the point of high arousal.

Get into the position: Sit in the center of the bed (or floor) facing each other. Wrap your legs around each other so that she is "sitting" on his legs. Place your right hand at the back of your lover's neck, your left hand on his or her tailbone.

Each presses the palm firmly at the base of the other's spine. Slide your hand up your lover's back to the base of his or her neck. Imagine that, as you slide your hand, you are channeling sexual energy up through your lover's body, warming him or her from the genitals, through the heart, and then through the head. Repeat the stroke over and over until you are both feeling very aroused.

Insert his penis into her vagina so that the shaft exerts as much indirect pressure as possible on her clitoris. While maintaining eye contact, rock slowly together as you rub each other's backs.

After her orgasm, make love in other positions, varying the speed, thrust, and angle of thrusting to prolong his excitation phase as long as possible.

....

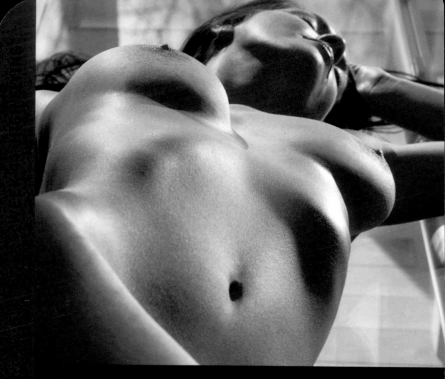

The Breast Stroke

Put your hands curved on her (fully clothed) breasts, palms over her nipples, fingers splayed. Press gently.

Raise your fingers and rub circles around her nipples with your palms.

Softly caress each breast as you kiss her and look into her eyes.

....

Movie Quickies #1: *Body Heat*

This movie is so hot that you never question why there appeared to be no air-conditioning in Florida in the late twentieth century. Odd. But William Hurt and Kathleen Turner in their sexual prime make questions irrelevant.

The hottest scene: He breaks the glass, turns the lock, and lets himself into the entryway of her house—while she watches. (Couldn't she open the door? Again, you don't question as you're watching.) He hikes her red pencil skirt up her thighs and takes her right there.

To re-create the scene without breaking glass:

Dressed in a pencil skirt, white shirt, no panties, and stiletto pumps, she is waiting for him when he comes home. He throws down his briefcase and takes her hungrily in his arms. She raises one leg, bent at the knee, and he pushes that skirt up, caressing her thigh. They kiss and fondle one another like animals in heat.

Pushing her skirt up to her waist, he grabs her into his arms and leans against the wall. The position gives him support so that he can hold her up with his hand under one buttock. Instead of wrapping her leg around his waist in the classic pose, she raises it, bent at the knee, as she did when he grabbed her inside the door. This gives her more clitoral stimulation and lets her feel his hot hand caressing her thigh.

He takes her fast and a little rough.

. . . .

The Urban BJ #2: The Fire Escape

It doesn't have to be your fire escape. Maybe you are walking down a deserted city street and spy a sturdy ladder to a fire escape on the side of a building. You notice that the shadows or nearby foliage provide cover. Take your man by the hand and tell him to put his hands over his head and hold on to the rung while you ravish him.

Cover his hands with yours so your body is flat against his. Bump and grind against him as you kiss him passionately.

When you feel his erection pushing insistently against you, unzip his pants and fondle it. Work his shaft with one hand as you continue to kiss him. Run your other hand through his hair and massage his chest.

Get down in a squatting position so that your head blocks the view of his penis in your mouth from a stray passerby.

Use the hand and mouth strokes that bring him to orgasm most quickly. Suction is generally a good closer.

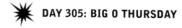

✳️ **DAY 305: BIG O THURSDAY**

His G-Spot Orgasm

You found his G-spot (page 66). If he responds to G-spot stimulation, he can probably have an orgasm that way. According to Lou Paget, massaging the prostate heightens three parts of the male orgasmic response:

1. The contractions and pulsing of the urethral bulb inside the prostate

2. The contractions of the prostate

3. The contractions of the PC muscle

There are two ways to get him there: external and internal G-spot massage.

External

1. He lies on his back; you are between his legs.

2. Hold his cock in one hand and massage his perineum with the other. Alternate pressing your thumb and circling your finger pads.

3. Use your knuckles.

4. Add a vibe. Tickle him with the ears of your Rabbit. Or use a small vibe, such as a bullet on low speed or a finger vibe.

Internal

1. Use a finger cot or latex glove and plenty of lube.

2. Insert your finger gently into his anus. (You can also use a slender anal vibe.)

3. Make the gentle "come hither" movement with your finger toward his belly button.

Stroke in and out slowly and gently, with your finger slightly curved (again toward his belly button).

....

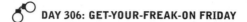

Taking It Out #2:
Sex Club/Sex Party Rules

Most big cities have a few sex clubs—some private, members only, some public, charging a fee at the door. Generally, couples and single women are welcome, but men alone are not. Condoms and single packets of lube are usually available on the premises. Rules are either posted or handed out on cards. You won't be forced to participate, but you will probably have to take off your clothes (or most of them).

Sex parties are hosted by groups of players who have developed clear rules of conduct that guests are expected to observe. Request the guidelines. Some parties permit sex acts short of intercourse. You can do almost anything at others as long as you are practicing safe sex. As in sex clubs, condoms and lube packets are usually available. No one should ever feel pressured into participating or "performing."

Palagia's OneLegUp parties, held at various venues in New York City, are high-end events attracting visiting Europeans and guests from all over the United States. Check out her website at OneLegUpNYC.com. First-timers can start with her "Take-Outs," the no-intercourse parties, and move up to "Eat-Ins."

There's sex and there's Sex. Have a program before heading out to a party or club. Many couples don't swing or participate in group sex. They get aroused by watching, go to a private corner, and have sex with one another only, their excitement fueled by what is happening around them.

....

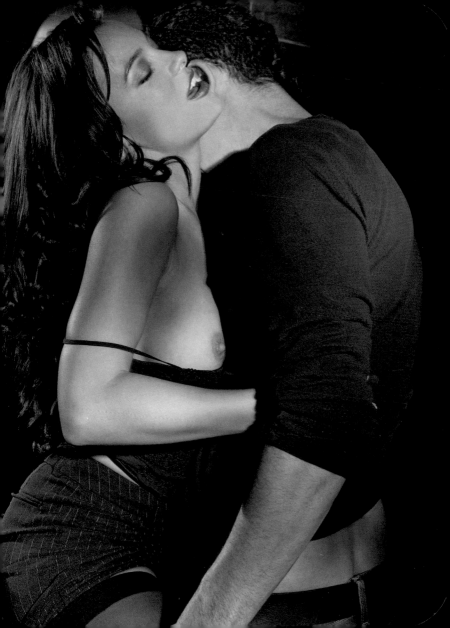

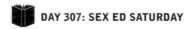

Dance Lessons #3: Dirty Dancing

Dirty Dancing, the 1987 film starring the late Patrick Swayze and Jennifer Gray, has one of, if not *the*, sexiest dance scenes in film history. The film spawned an oldies music revival and dance floors full of dirty dancers. Almost twenty-five years later, the film, the music, and the dancing hold up.

Watch *Dirty Dancing* together. Get the soundtrack.

Go back to the scene where Jennifer's character, Baby, gets her first dirty dancing lesson. Watch closely, then get your bodies into the same groove.

Incorporate dirty dancing moves into your sex play—for example, thrusting pelvises in a full-body hug.

Switch up your sex routine by making dirty dancing your foreplay tonight.

....

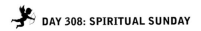 **DAY 308: SPIRITUAL SUNDAY**

The Passion Flower Position

I created this position for *Redbook* magazine to meet their three criteria: greater intimacy than most intercourse positions for her, longer-lasting state of high arousal for him, and exceptional orgasms for both. The Passion Flower, an adaptation of the classic Yab-Yum (page 361), proved popular with both testers and readers.

Sit in the center of your bed facing each other. His legs can be straight out or bent at the knees. Wrap her legs comfortably around his body so that she is sitting on his thighs.

Each places his or her right hand at the base of the other's neck and left hand at the base of the spine. Caress each other's necks and stroke up each other's backs. Eye gaze and kiss with open eyes.

Insert his erect penis into her vagina so that the shaft exerts as much indirect pressure on her clitoris as possible. Rock together, slowly rubbing backs and kissing. Because of the intense clitoral stimulation the position provides, she should be able to reach orgasm this way, while the lack of deep thrusting helps him sustain intercourse.

After her first orgasm, they can move into one of their favorite positions affording more vigorous thrusting.

. . . .

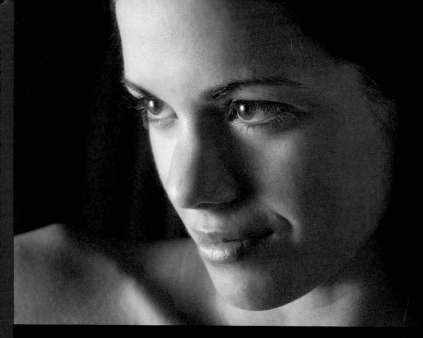

DAY 309: FLIRTATION AND FOREPLAY MONDAY

Lick Your Lover's Lips

Offer him a taste of something. If you are not likely to be in front of the stove stirring a sauce with a wooden spoon, pull something out of the refrigerator, such as a jar of fudge sauce or jam. As you give him a taste, smear a little bit on his lips.

Hold his face in your hands. Using the tip of your tongue, lick his lips clean. Press your lips against his. Look deeply into his eyes. Now pull away.

....

Movie Quickies #2: *The English Patient*

One of my all-time favorite films, *The English Patient*, won Best Picture of 1996 and eight other Oscars at the Academy Awards the following year. Based on the equally wonderful novel by Michael Ondaatje, the film, set toward the end of World War II, starred Ralph Fiennes and Kristin Scott-Thomas as the doomed adulterous lovers. The sex was intense and entirely believable.

In my favorite scene, she is in his bathtub. You can see the steam rising from between her thighs. They fucked until exhausted but not sated. And his obsession with her is obvious.

Watch *The English Patient* together in bed.

If you get through it without having sex—which I doubt you will—go into the bathroom anyway.

He draws a hot bath for her. She leans back in the water, her legs open (because they are chafed), while he squeezes water from a bath sponge onto her breasts.

They didn't have waterproof vibes in the 1940s, but don't let that stop you. Bring her to orgasm in the tub.

. . . .

The Urban CJ #2: The Fire Escape

For many city dwellers, the fire escape is their little patch of "outdoors." Although strictly speaking it's illegal, people put their plants out to catch the sun (or rain) and set up their mini grills to fix a steak or two. Why not a fire escape CJ?

Wear a skirt, no panties. Put a blanket or rug on the fire escape platform. Climb out your window. Sit facing it, with your legs open, knees bent, or with your legs inside the window. (You live in a condo or house with a real deck or patio? Sit on a chaise lounge or the steps.)

Draping your skirt over his head, he uses the hand and mouth strokes that bring you to orgasm quickly. Tell him what you want. ("Lick my clit," "Put your lips around it and pucker," etc.) The dirty talk in public will heighten the excitement for both of you.

Since he can't see your face, direct him by the pressure of your hands on his head.

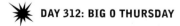

✴ **DAY 312: BIG O THURSDAY**

The Bigger O Trick #1: In Your Hands

The problematic nature of female orgasm is the big engine driving every sex philosophy, therapy, and theory. Yet the very first step a woman needs to take is rarely discussed. She can get advice on how to have anal intercourse—but probably not masturbation!—in a mainstream women's magazine.

The most important message we should be giving young women is: **masturbate**.

If a woman has never masturbated, how likely is it that she knows how she reaches orgasm? Not very. She's depending on her partner and serendipity to get her there when the truth would set her free.

Women like sex better when they reach orgasm often, and that's not going to happen for most women without direct clitoral stimulation. Masturbating regularly:

- Makes her more comfortable touching herself with a partner

- Teaches her what she needs to know about her body's responses to make orgasm happen in partner sex

- Encourages sexual confidence

- Takes the pressure off her partner to "make" her come or "give" her an orgasm

- Makes her a more relaxed, vibrant, and healthier person

Partnered or unpartnered, every woman needs to masturbate. I believe she should own a wardrobe of vibes and give herself an orgasm with one daily. Dr. Ruth says that a sexpert is a permission giver. You have mine. Go play.

....

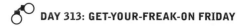

Bringing It In: Your Private Party Rules

Do you secretly yearn to be one of those suburban couples hosting sex parties? (Order *The Ice Storm* from Netflix. You will be both titillated and very afraid.) Before you issue invitations, create your party rules.

Some suggestions:

1. Agree on who is invited—only couples, couples plus single women, couples plus singles of both genders?

2. Decide in advance whether you're hosting a cuddle party, a limited sex acts party, or an all-out orgy. (Hint: Start modestly.)

3. Set a limit for number of guests.

4. On your invitations, be clear on neighborhood rules regarding parking, noise, drinking outside, etc.

5. Be clear on house rules, such as whether you will allow smoking, marijuana, or other recreational drugs; most important, specify that "No" means no and safer sex practices must be instituted if it's a full-on sex party. Will people be asked to leave if they are drinking too heavily? Or putting pressure on other guests? Spell it all out. Enforce the rules.

....

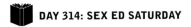

Dance Lessons #4: Tango

There is a definite connection between music and sex—and the connection is never stronger than in tango.

Tango was born in the Buenos Aires brothels in the mid-1800s and spread to the cities of Europe, with Paris leading the first international Tango craze in 1912. Wealthy Argentines didn't embrace their native dance until it was a success abroad.

But Tantra Tango, created by Richard Anton Diaz, World Champion Latin Ballroom Dancer and Tantra teacher, is an even sexier tango that "fuses the energies of Tantra with the dark, intimate dance of the tango." Introducing the Tantric element, Diaz says, "deepens connections that allow us to dance intimately with a stranger. My desire to teach this most sensual social dance was in large part inspired by my lonely nights as bachelor, when I got my 'fix' for intimacy and affection by simply going out to a tango salon. There I had the opportunity to be in close embrace with many women in one evening, their breasts pressed against my chest, our eyes closed inward as if making secret love. I went home alone, as desired, but felt so fulfilled from my intimate connections with women who, to this day, I don't even know."

Take tango lessons, and then go out and dance with strangers before you dance together.

....

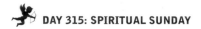 **DAY 315: SPIRITUAL SUNDAY**

Spiritual Sex and Religion

Scholars of religion, spirituality, and sexuality tell me that it is possible to be intensely spiritual and sexual at the same time. That seems like a contradiction to many of us because we live in a culture where organized religion is typically sexually repressive. Thomas Moore, author of *The Soul of Sex* says, "If a person's sexuality is not fully accepted, his spirituality will suffer. And vice versa: If his spirituality is not strong, his sexuality will be weak."

Many modern lovers are heeding his words. Whether you consider yourself "spiritual" or not, you can have better sex by tapping into the spirit part of the body/mind/spirit equation. Without realizing it, you've been developing your spiritual sexual side by defining and redefining "sex."

According to Moore, we become more spiritual as we deepen our sexual experience—and vice versa. The Sufi teachers often say that your ultimate lover is God. That may be taking it further than most of us are willing to go. Today, reflect on what the words *spiritual*, *sexual*, and *religious* mean to you. Read spiritual/sexual writings to one another.

The Soul of Sex by Thomas Moore

The Art of Sexual Ecstasy by Margot Anand

Taoist Secrets of Love by Mantak Chia

Passionate Enlightenment by Miranda Shaw

Spiritual Sex by Nik Douglas

....

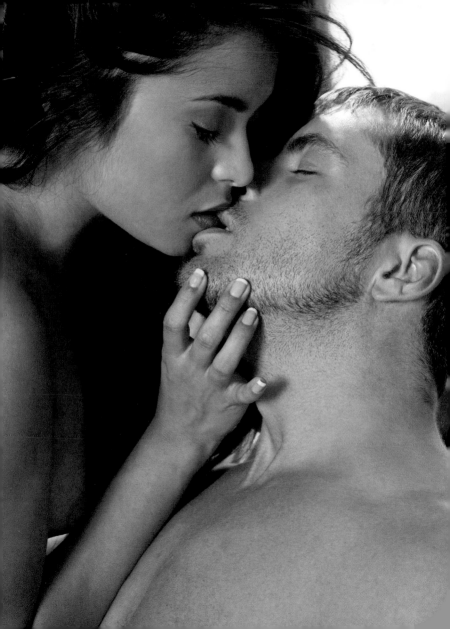

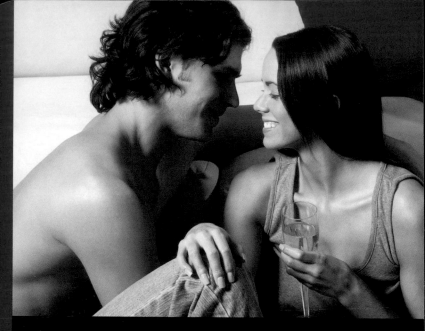

The Temple Massage

She's had a tough day, and she's tense. (Or he has, and he is.) Envelope her in your arms and hold her. No hugging or pressing of your body against hers. Just hold.

Remain standing close and, with the first two fingers of both hands, massage her temples. Move your fingers in circles, pressing gently, then with a slight increase in pressure and back to softer pressure.

Kiss her forehead.

. . . .

Movie Quickies #3: *Bull Durham*

Susan Sarandon is a sexual presence on screen, no matter what film she's in—except maybe the nun in *Dead Man Walking*. As the highly sexed fan of a minor league baseball team in *Bull Durham*, she sizzled. My favorite scene is really the montage of her and Kevin Costner toward the end of the film. They make *love*. And there's a bathtub and lots of candles . . .

Light some candles, turn out the lights, and watch the film together in bed.

As you snuggle up to your lover, touch his (her) body in long, tender, loving strokes. Make every touch a lingering one.

After this sustained romantic movie foreplay, get on top of your man. With Sarandon as your role model, what other position would feel right?

. . . .

The Suburban BJ #2: The Tree House

A SexyPrime reader sent this BJ tip and erotic anecdote centered around the tree house his father built for him.

My wife and I took care of putting my parents' home on the market after he went off to assisted living. We were walking the property and I said, "Look, the old tree house; let's climb up."

(continued on next page)

I went up first. Coming up the ladder behind me, she bit my ass and said, "Pull down your shorts and get on your back!" I thought she was going to get on top of me, but she knelt between my legs, took my cock in her expert hands, and rubbed it between them as if she were building a fire. She rubbed for a little while after she took the head in her mouth and began to suck. Her hands played jazz on my shaft and testicles while her tongue and lips kept their own beat.

Suddenly I was a horny kid, jerking off and dreaming about this. She sucked me dry and I was a man again, renewed and restored.

....

 DAY 319: BIG O THURSDAY

The Bigger O Trick #2:
Eyes Open/Eyes Closed

Women *can* learn to separate love and sex. It's a necessary skill—for married women as well as single—as necessary as the opposite skill, being able to create an intimate sexual experience. Eyes open soul gazing is not the only way to have sex with your partner. But who tells you that?

Eyes open when—

• You are feeling solidly connected to one another.

• You want to know and feel known.

• You want to see your lover's pleasure.

Eyes closed when—

- You ask yourself, Who is he/she and why did I marry him/her?

- You would rather not share your thoughts and feelings.

- You want to focus on your own pleasure.

If you are angry with each other, he likely still wants to have sex. You don't. Maybe he sees sex as the way to make up, or maybe he just wants sex. Transform your anger into passion. Close your eyes and do it in rear-entry position. Fantasize about another man. Enjoy the sex. The bonus: You won't be so mad at each other afterward. Orgasms make people feel grateful.

············

 DAY 320: GET-YOUR-FREAK-ON FRIDAY

Sexual Truth or Dare

This was just a kid's game until Madonna gave it edge in a documentary about her touring life. Can you play on her level?

The rules are simple. You take turns giving one another the opportunity to tell a previously untold truth—or accept the dare. Pull out the toy and costume boxes. Props will surely be involved.

Some suggestions for truth questions or dares:

- Show me how you kissed your first girlfriend.

- Have you ever masturbated while I was asleep?

- Let me pick the costume for you to wear to take the trash bins out to the street.

- What's the dirtiest thing you've ever fantasized doing to me? Or me to you?

- Do twenty naked push-ups with an erection.

- Have you ever put on the nipple clamps when you were home alone?

- Give me a lap dance and shake your booty in my face.

- Did a man ever call you on faking an orgasm?

- Pick a historical character and show me how she/he masturbates.

- What is your hidden sexual desire?

....

 DAY 321: SEX ED SATURDAY

A Tutorial in Classic Porn

Steve Otero, cofounder of Sexy Spirits, is widely regarded in the sex world (my name for the sex research/adult education/product sales/entertainment industry) as the man who knows where to find the answers. He is a walking catalog of background information on everything from sex education seminars being taught anywhere in the country to the current thinking (from all perspectives) on sex addiction, and anything else you can think to ask him. If it's a sex topic, he's on it. He knows classic porn like nobody else.

Steve and I both lament the decline of good porn. (Isn't everybody tired of tight penetration shots in all three female orifices?) Here are his picks.

The Top Five Porn Films of All Time

1. *The Opening of Misty Beethoven*, 1976, directed by Radley Metzger (a.k.a. Henry Paris), with Jamie Gillis and Constance Money. Still after all these years the best produced porn film of all time. Just watch it.

2. *The Devil in Miss Jones*, 1973, directed by Gerard Damiano, with Georgina Spelvin. The tragedy of sexual repression, ecstasy, and eternal loneliness.

3. *Behind the Green Door*, 1972, directed by Artie and Jim Mitchell, with Marilyn Chambers. The debut of Goddess Marilyn.

4. *Hard Edge*, 2003, directed by Andrew Blake, filmed on location in Paris. Bold, uninhibited, raw erotic tension, where fantasy and reality collide.

5. *Dog Walker*, 1995, directed by John Leslie. Funded by Leslie using his own money, shot on film, jazzy blues score. Raw, hot sex!

. . . .

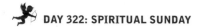 **DAY 322: SPIRITUAL SUNDAY**

The New Commandments

Read these aloud to one another and commit to keeping the erotic commandments alive in your spiritual sex life.

The Ten Erotic Commandments (according to Thomas Moore)

1. Ethics—Treat your partner honestly, respectfully, and kindly. It's as simple as that.

2. Partnership—Sex is a union of persons, not only bodies.

3. Vision—A spiritual person has a broad transcendent vision, beyond self.

4. Contemplation—Steady, calm progress to a state that is tranquil and otherworldly.

5. Ritual—The sacred habits of sex (see Spiritual Sundays).

6. Generosity—The great virtue in sex.

7. Beauty—Sex has a lot to do with appreciating the beauty of the human body and the person.

8. Prayer—Prayer takes many forms.

9. Devotion—To one another and to your sexuality.

10. Community—Spirituality involves reaching beyond the self. Sex is quite private, but a good sex life can help make a good community.

....

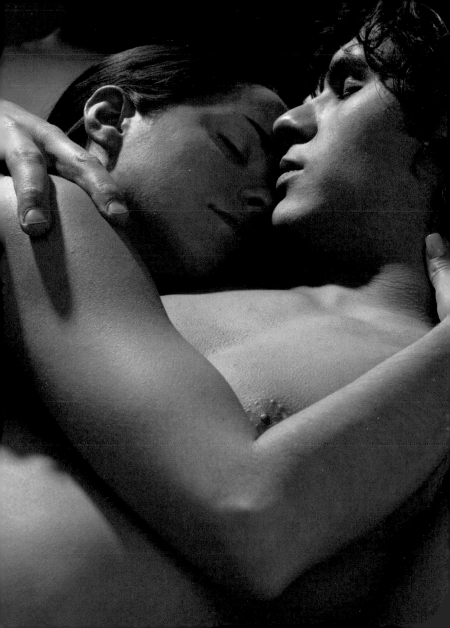

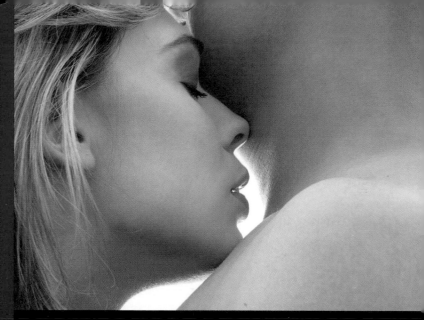

DAY 323: FLIRTATION AND FOREPLAY MONDAY

The Eyelid Kiss

Take your lover's face in your hands. Kiss her (or him) softly. If her eyes are open, take one finger and ever so gently close them. Press your lips against her closed eyelids, one at a time.

Hold her in your arms and whisper, "I love you."

. . . .

Movie Quickies #4: *Unfaithful*

Film as foreplay. It's easy, fun, and so relaxing. No pressure. You lie in bed together, watching the movie, perhaps drifting in and out of sleep and slipping in and out of erotic contact. Stroke, kiss, doze—and suddenly the sexy part has you.

Unfaithful, which came out in 2002, is Diane Lane's movie. Richard Gere plays her husband and Olivier Martinez, her lover—but it's her sexiest film. In her first illicit sex scene, she sways her hips to African music in a Soho apartment. Frightened by the intensity of her desire for a stranger, she runs out—but runs back because she's forgotten her coat. A shot of her naked in his bed, her belly trembling as he touches her thighs, is so arouslng, you forget to breathe.

As you're watching the film, imagine what it would feel like to be the cheating wife or the cuckolded husband. Play with those ideas in your mind. Let the tension build.

Tease each other with unfamiliar strokes. If he does not usually lick her inner thighs or her instep or pull her hair, he should do these things now. Come together in an intense kiss, your interisity fueled by the fantasy of being caught in a love triangle.

....

Oral Sex Positions

Just as you change coital dynamics by switching intercourse positions, you can create new sensations from the familiar strokes of oral sex by varying your position.

- On Your Knees, the classic fellatio pose (and my favorite), also works for cunnilingus. Hands free all around. Put a pillow under your knees and it's perfect.

- Lying Between Legs is the classic cunnilingus position. You can work with it by putting her legs on his shoulders, bending her knees, or leaving her legs flat.

- Sitting on Face, for him or her, puts the receiver in control and provides full range of motion.

- Right Angles, where the giver kneels at the side of the receiver, who is lying flat, gives him access to more of her body, including her breasts and nipples.

- On the Edge of the Chair is basically On Your Knees, but with the receiver's genitals closer to the giver's mouth. It's the preferred position for servicing the boss from under the desk.

....

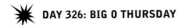 **DAY 326: BIG O THURSDAY**

The Magic of Ten

Corey Silverberg is About.com's sexuality editor. I thoroughly enjoy his weekly newsletter and usually learn something I didn't know. This is his advice to readers on how to slow down their orgasms to create greater intensity. It's a little different than the techniques you've learned here and definitely worth trying.

Find Your Line, Then Mess with It

Don't be in such a hurry to get to orgasm that you lose the buildup. If you can always tell when you're going to come, you can watch the signs and "mess with your line."

Prolong the period just before orgasm by masturbating to the brink and then slowing down. Don't stop stimulation, but "step back from the line."

Repeat the move three or four times before letting yourself come.

After some practice, you may be able to do this ten times, for an orgasm that is "The Magic of Ten."

....

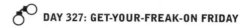

The Cum Shot #1:
Ejaculating on Breasts

I've said this before: If he wants to re-create a porn scene, the cum shots are the easiest. Some women say they feel "degraded" by having a man come on their body. But have they tried it? Many women agree with me that it's a playful experience, like body painting or licking honey dust.

Some men (generally younger) ejaculate further than others. His "shooting distance" is a factor in setting up the shot.

Have your cell phone or other mini cam ready. Positioning the camera for an "up and under" (looking up from the underside of the shaft) will make his penis appear larger and his distance more impressive. When he is near ejaculation, let him pull out and come on your breasts. Snap several shots.

....

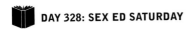

DAY 328: SEX ED SATURDAY

Fusion Tantra Position #1:
The Moving Sit

This position is from my book *The New Tantra: Simple and Sexy* and is adapted from the Tantra Rocking Horse, which allows sexual energy to build slowly and gives him an intimate view of her vagina.

1. He sits with his legs open wide; she sits between his legs, facing him.

2. He clasps her wrists or forearms to support her as she puts one leg over his shoulder.

3. She leans back as he penetrates her, resting her weight on her outstretched arms.

4. They move together gently until both are highly aroused.

5. She lowers her leg from his shoulder and wraps both ankles around his body at chest level.

6. They rock back and forth while clasping one another's wrists and forearms.

. . . .

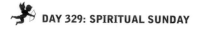 **DAY 329: SPIRITUAL SUNDAY**

Sexual/Spiritual Gender Roles

Tantra is a Sanskrit word for an Eastern spiritual and sexual philosophy that emphasizes experiential approaches to life and lovemaking. The word *tantra* has various translations, including "weaving." Weaving together male (represented by the Hindu god Shiva) and female (the Hindu goddess Shakti), Tantra unifies not only man and woman as lovers, but also the male and female elements within each of us.

Yes, the concept is similar to the Taoist/Buddhist yin and yang. Ancient philosophies were in many ways more sophisticated in addressing the sexual and spiritual roles of gender than we are today. Books and magazine articles posit theories about whether the alpha male is declining and what that means to the relationship between the sexes now that a significant number of women, 30 percent or more, outearn their husbands, who are relegated to the category of beta male. And I have been asking on SexyPrime: "What does the new economic relationship dynamic mean to men and women in their sex lives?"

Put that question up for debate today. You can find examples in Hindu and Taoist mythology of strong men *and* strong women, just as you can in the world you live in. Often the strongest, bravest, and boldest heroes and heroines were also the most capable of emotional vulnerability.

How would you describe each other's and your own elements of strength and vulnerability in your sex life?

....

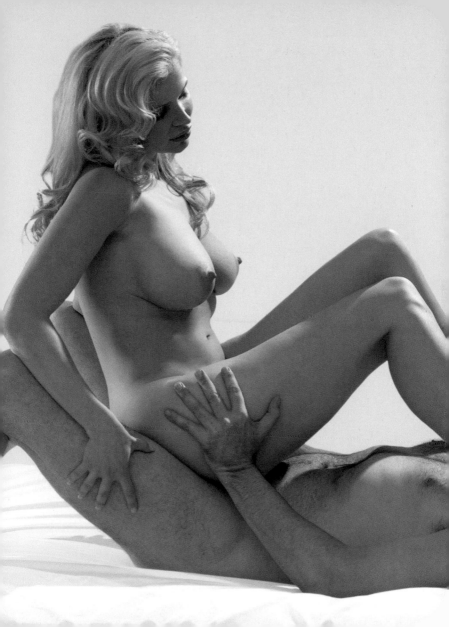

DAY 330: FLIRTATION AND FOREPLAY MONDAY

The Naked Surprise

Couples who have been together a while are rarely surprised by seeing one another nude. Yet a naked surprise is so titillating. Catch your partner off guard and show it off.

Some suggestions:

- Streak through the family room while he's watching TV.

- Meet her at the door wearing a shirt and socks, no pants.

- Send him out to the garage or down to the basement on an errand—and get naked from the waist down.

- When you're dining home alone, serve dinner partially clothed.

- Do your weight routine naked (pages 188 and 196).

- Pull down your pants and moon her on the way out the door.

....

The Rough Touch Quickie

Almost everybody likes it rough occasionally. Take him—and make him like it. Turn him on by hot kisses and firm hands on his body.

1. He lies on his back; she is on top.

2. Lean forward and pinch or bite his nipples. Squeeze his buttocks.

3. When he is highly aroused, create a pause in the coital dynamics by clenching your PC and squeezing his penis tightly.

4. Release. Thrust up and down (while stimulating your clitoris). Use your PC muscle again to control the thrusting and pull him in deeper.

5. When he is close to orgasm, make intense eye contact with him and pinch his nipples as he comes.

. . . .

The Historical BJ #5:
Elizabeth I's Sir Walter Raleigh Special

The Tudors were a sexual clan. (If you are not yet a fan of the Showtime series *The Tudors,* catch up on DVD.) Elizabeth I, daughter of Henry VIII, was sometimes called the Virgin Queen because she did not marry,

(continued on next page)

a calculated decision to bolster her power. During the Elizabethan Age, arts and culture thrived, and apparently so did Elizabeth's libido. She was reputed to have had sex with men without removing her clothes. Historians of the day reported that she knelt before Sir Walter Raleigh, and then demanded privacy for the two of them. What would bring a queen to her knees? A royal blow job, of course.

After your man has greeted you with deference and respect, kneel before him.

Unzip his trousers and remove his splendid cock and the royal jewels. Lower your face to them, and press your lips against the shaft. Warm his balls in your mouth as you run your fingers lovingly up and down the shaft of his penis.

"Nibble" his shaft with teeth covered by lips. "Bite" the head of his penis in the same way.

Holding the base firmly in one hand, lick in long strokes up and down the shaft.

Take the head into your mouth and gently suck. Suck the first third of the shaft. Repeat the sucking moves, finishing them off by swirling the head with the tip of your tongue. Alternate sucking with strumming the frenulum and flicking the corona. Return to sucking.

Pick up the pace. When he is near orgasm, swallow him as deeply as you can.

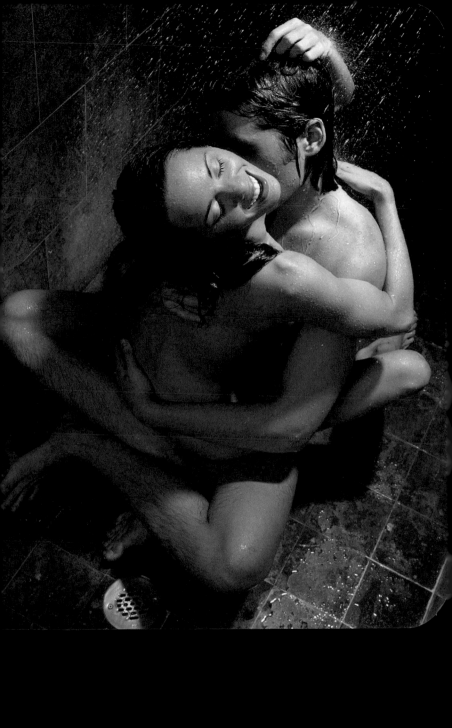

✸ **DAY 333: BIG O THURSDAY**

The Rule-of-Thumb Orgasm

Are you ready for another opinion on why most women don't reach orgasm on intercourse alone? Kim Wallen, professor of psychology and behavioral neuroendocrinology at Emory University, says, "Whether a woman has an orgasm during intercourse or not depends on how far her clitoris lies from her vagina."

The Rule-of-Thumb: Women with clitoris-vagina distances less than 1 inch (2.5 cm)—that's roughly from the tip of your thumb to your first knuckle—can reach orgasm during intercourse with no clitoral stimulation. More than a thumb's length? You need a helping hand or vibe.

Wallen is re-creating the research of Princess Marie Bonaparte, a French psychoanalyst and close friend of Sigmund Freud, who collected C-V orgasm data in the 1920s. Rejecting the term *frigid*, she looked for answers to her own and her patients' lack of orgasmic response.

Wallen's research seems to support the prevailing theory: It's all about the clitoris, including the hidden parts of it behind the vaginal wall.

Have him measure your C-V distance—and continue playing researcher as he brings you to oral and manual orgasms.

. . . .

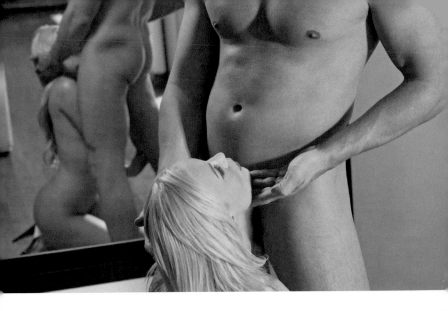

 DAY 334: GET-YOUR-FREAK-ON FRIDAY

The Cum Shot #2: Giving Her Pearls

Get your camera ready for his second set of cum shots. Have him straddle your face with your head thrown back, the better to show off your pearls when he gives them to you.

Using a combination of favorite BJ strokes, bring him to the verge of orgasm.

He pulls out, holds his cock, and directs his ejaculate so that it forms a string of pearls around your neck, while you are catching him on your cell phone or other small camera.

. . . .

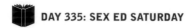

The Gentle Chinese Sex Position: The Wedding Night

According to legend, Chinese husbands in the period of the Ming dynasty put their young virginal brides in this position so that the more shallow penetration would ease deflowering. It's also nice when a woman is feeling tired or fragile, physically or emotionally.

1. She lies on her back with her hips at the edge of the bed, her legs hung over the sides, feet on the floor.

2. He stands in front of her and leans into her between her parted legs.

3. As he enters her, he caresses her buttocks and thighs. He leans his body over hers and strokes her clitoris while thrusting.

4. The position is instantly adaptable to accommodate a sudden change of mood. If she feels suddenly energetic, she can create leverage with her feet on the floor or wrap her legs around his waist or put them up on his shoulders.

5. In a variation, she, no longer the shy bride, lies face down, her legs over the edge of the bed as before. He can hold up her thighs as he enters from the rear.

....

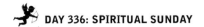

DAY 336: SPIRITUAL SUNDAY

How Much Do You Love Her Pussy/His Cock?

I occasionally run surveys on SexyPrime. The two most popular have been the Penis Survey and the Vulva Survey. Each had a man's version and a woman's. Although I was interested to learn how readers relate to their own genitals, I was awestruck at the love many men have for the pussy and many women for the cock. It's a beautiful thing.

Love the pussy, big-time. If you love the pussy right, a woman will beg to do things to you that you will like a whole lot, or sometimes just grab on and do them without waiting to ask. Unlike post-orgasmic guys who have that lamentable tendency to just fall asleep, post-orgasmic women are often energized, very excited, and not nearly ready to stop. "Ladies first" really works and most women love it, appreciate what you're doing, and show that appreciation. Selflessness can be selfish, I suppose, but good giving usually means great getting.

If I weren't empowered sexually, I wouldn't be able to admit how much I adore the cock. I love the shape and size—the heft of a solid appendage held in my hand—and the texture of the skin, the silkiness of the shaft, the lush spongy head. I love the smell and the feel of it in my hands, my mouth, my vagina (yes, and occasionally, my anus, too). I love what I can do to that cock, how I can make it perform beyond his expectations and derive more pleasure for both of us than he thought possible. The cock— better than a magic carpet ride. What magic carpet ever came with broad shoulders, strong arms and legs, and chest hair?

....

Stroke Her with a Flower

"This was what she missed as much as the sex: the flattery. In the early throes of love, you complimented each other. Then you got married and spent the rest of your years hurling insults and complaints. Marriage was disappointment verbalized."

—From *Prospect Park West* by Amy Sohn.

This is the sort of thing she is reading in her book club. Novels have long chronicled women's disenchantment with marriage and the loss of romance it represents.

Buy her flowers today for no reason. Take one from the bunch that you hand her. Stroke her face with the bloom and tell her as she exclaims over the flowers, "They are not as beautiful as you are."

....

The Remote-Control Quickie

She's not responsible for her own quickie arousal today. He is. But he can't touch her with any part of his body to drive her so wild she's begging him to take her *now*.

Get out the remote-controlled vibe. (The panty vibes are ultra-discreet.)

Tease her by starting/stopping stimulation.

If she looks like she's ready to vibrate to orgasm on high, turn it back to low or stop briefly.

When she begs, pull her onto your lap for a sitting quickie.

This is the perfect quickie for the night he brings work home but she wants to play.

....

The Faux Deep Throat

Combine these two moves for the Faux Deep Throat:

Lou Paget's the Ring and the Seal

Form a ring with your thumb and fingers. Attach it to your mouth and hold it there as you perform fellatio. The Ring and the Seal effectively "lengthens" your mouth, meaning you will take less of his cock into it.

Dr. Sonia Borg's the Faux Deep Throat

When he is thrusting too vigorously into your mouth and his orgasm is imminent, flatten your tongue to the roof of your mouth, creating the sensation that he is going down your throat when he is really going to the back of your tongue.

....

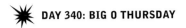

The Multi-Position Orgasm

Sometimes both partners can get a bigger orgasm by changing intercourse positions several times and rapidly. This is different than alternating stimuli, where he stops thrusting and gives her oral or manual stimulation. It's fast, furious, and hot. A memorable SexyPrime post:

He pulled a packet of silky lubricant from his nightstand and massaged it around my clit, into my labia, and then swirled a generous finger-full inside my vagina. He knelt between my legs, took his lovely erection into his hand, and teased the tip and sides of my clit. I moved toward him; he pulled back. He stroked my labia with the head of his penis and returned to the clit, bringing my arousal up slowly.

But I can only be teased by the head of a penis for so long before my sex nerve endings are screaming for more. I wrapped one leg around his waist, pulling him inside me. He thrust deep, hard, and fast for a few strokes, simultaneously playing with my clit and giving me the first orgasm, and then eased up. Under his deft direction, we moved from this open missionary position—with my other leg remaining bent, foot on the bed—into the female superior, the reverse cowgirl, and finally back to the missionary with both legs wrapped around his waist as he drove his orgasm home. Oh, yes, it was good!

I can't believe that I once thought his athletic management of multiple positions per session was turning sex into a bit of an amateur Olympics event. What was I thinking? It's the specialty of the house.

....

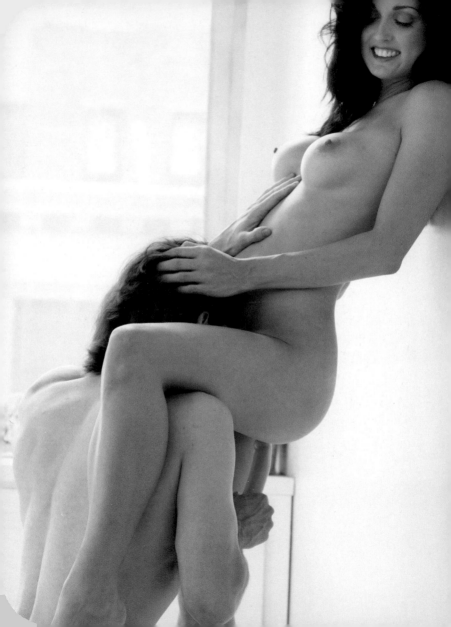

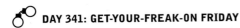

DAY 341: GET-YOUR-FREAK-ON FRIDAY

Just DO IT

Men's most common sex complaint is frequency. They report they aren't getting enough. (In fact, cheating husbands use it as their number one excuse/justification.)

Women complain almost as much about frequency. In the alpha woman/ beta male marriage, he is often the one with the headache.

And several times a week someone emails me on SexyPrime, asking: What can I do to make my sex life hotter immediately?

The answer is obvious. You can't get hotter if you aren't even getting warm. So, JUST SAY "YES!"

Don't be too tired, too stressed, too busy, too worried about your job, the bills, the kids' grades. Say "Yes." (Men, the same advice applies to you.)

If your partner is the naysayer, counter that with: "What do you want? I'll give it to you. Oral sex? Come on my face? A little anal play? Spank me? I spank you? Bend me over the deck railing? Tell me what you want; I'm ready to deal."

Deal. Make something happen tonight.

. . . .

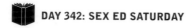

Sex Online

A recent study conducted by the University of Sydney in Australia found that 70 percent of men watch porn online while only 30 percent of women do. Watching porn in moderation is a healthy expression of sexuality with no harmful effects. (But porn shouldn't be a man's only form of sex education.) If he'd rather masturbate to porn than have sex with the woman in his bed, then porn does become a relationship issue.

Make online porn a couples' viewing experience today.

Some suggestions:

- YouPorn is the world's #1 website. Check out the videos of real people having real sex. You may laugh, you may be disgusted, and you may get turned on.

- Avoid the misogynist, hardest-core porn. Even nice guys will occasionally look at it, but few women will want to know that. The viewing experience could devolve into "but how can you watch that horrible stuff?"

- Let her choose what you will watch for longer than a few minutes.

....

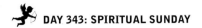 **DAY 343: SPIRITUAL SUNDAY**

The Sexual Puja

Animals have been worshipped in many religions and cultures throughout history. The Hindus, for example, revere Hanuman, the monkey god; Ganesha, the boy with an elephant's head; and others. Egyptians worshipped the cat. Aided by strong wine, they also danced to a sexual frenzy in celebration of snakes.

Our culture's cat is a cougar. No matter what your age, you can play at being a big cat.

Tease him by flashing your genitals at him before you undress slowly. If he isn't hard, suck his cock long enough to get him there. Push your man down on his back and straddle him, assume a prowling stance, and kneel on all fours over him with your knees near his hips. Use your claws lightly and sparingly on his thighs as you lower your face and breasts to his chest, grazing his nipples with yours. Purr while you lick and gently bite his chest, neck, and finally his lips. Circle your tongue around his as you continue to hold him down.

Spread your legs wider so your hips are near his and your vagina touches his penis. Move your hips back and forth, rubbing your labia on his shaft to arouse him and to stimulate your clitoris. Guide his penis into your vagina with one hand. Keep the other on his shoulder, holding him down.

After a few moments of intercourse, climb off him, leaving him begging for more. Tease him by rubbing your body against his. Resume intercourse. (By interrupting your lovemaking with more cat play, you help him delay ejaculation, making his orgasm feel stronger.)

. . . .

DAY 344: FLIRTATION AND FOREPLAY MONDAY

Give Him a Cigar

A beautiful and quite successful Manhattan call girl recently told me that she carries a good Cuban cigar in her bag when she meets wealthy clients. Why? Many men want the "presidential cigar"—so named because Monica Lewinsky reputedly held a cigar in her vagina before offering it to the President Clinton.

"You might think that only older guys, the aging boomers, want the special cigar—but just as many young men do," she says.

While the client watches, she removes the cigar from her bag, unwraps it, and puts it inside her vagina. (She may do this before sex, but usually after, depending on the client's pleasure.) After it's been seasoned— "long enough to drink a glass of wine"—she takes it out, puts it in the client's mouth, and lights it for him.

....

The Scent Kiss Quickie

Do you wear a fragrance that really turns him on? Take that scent and use it as his road map to a hot quickie.

Bathe or shower. Perfume only the parts of your body that you want your lover to touch or kiss. These may be the obvious places, such as your wrists and neck, or those places where you secretly wish he would touch more often, such as the armpits, the backs of your knees, or inside the elbows.

Pick a vibe, one for either clitoral stimulation only or insertion, such as the rabbit. The vibe you choose will let him know whether you want an oral or an intercourse quickie. Spray a little fragrance on the part of a vibe that won't touch your clitoris or vagina.

Have him sniff lightly to find the scent on your body and then inhale deeply only those perfumed places. Ask him to kiss you there.

Now let him sniff your vibe.

. . . .

Out of the "She Comes First" Rut

Many men consider cunnilingus the way to give her an orgasm before intercourse, when they get theirs. That philosophy, popularized by the boomers led Dr. Ian Kerner to write two excellent books, *She Comes First* and *He Comes Next*. But even a steady diet of steak and lobster would be a rut. This is a sexual rut.

Two quick routes out of the "She Comes First" rut:

- Cunnilingus as extreme foreplay. Withdraw your tongue before she comes. Give her that orgasm during intercourse, when you have yours. Use either your hand or a finger vibe to stimulate her clitoris as you thrust.

- Another way to look at cunnilingus—you come too, while you're performing it. Put a vibrating bullet inside your pants or insert a vibrating butt plug or both. Pay attention to her responses as you lick and suck her. As her flesh pulsates and throbs in your mouth, imagine those sensations traveling throughout your body. Feel her moans and signs of pleasure deep inside your cock. Let her arousal ignite your own. Give yourself a few strokes, and you will come, too.

....

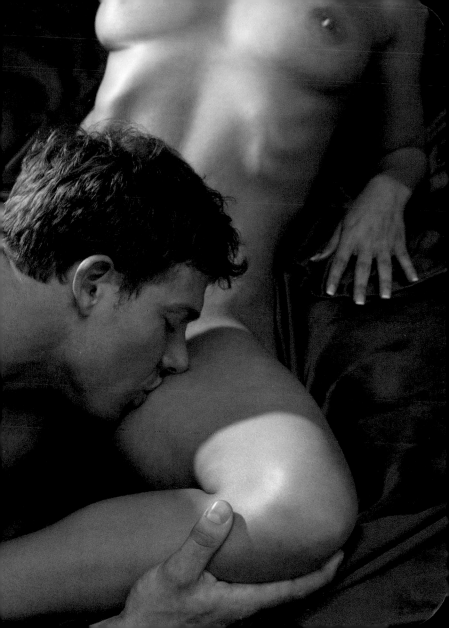

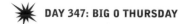

DAY 347: BIG O THURSDAY

Fusion Tantra Position #2:
Washer/Dryer Variation

Put more power into the spin cycle. She opens her legs as wide as she comfortably can, while sitting on the washer/dryer. He holds on to her hips, enters her, and thrusts vigorously. Her wide angle facilitates G-spot stimulation, and, of course, her hands are free to stimulate her clitoris.

Tantric bonus: intense eye contact in this face-to-face position.

Simple? Yes. But opening those legs wider makes a big difference.

. . . .

DAY 348: GET-YOUR-FREAK-ON FRIDAY

Strip Poker

Even if you played it once or twice at a party in college, you haven't played strip poker by these rules. The game changes when one partner is naked, turning into prolonged seduction poker. (Everybody wins.)

Start playing by the classic rules: one item of clothing for every lost hand. When one partner is naked, the rules change.

The loser of a hand must perform whatever sex act the other requests for two minutes—and only two minutes.

Play as long as you can. Then throw down the cards and do it.

. . . .

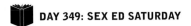 **DAY 349: SEX ED SATURDAY**

Lord Yang and Lady Yin—Cross-Dressing

If you want to find the yin in his yang and the yang in her yin, then play at cross-dressing. Do you have the courage for it?

Thor, the Germanic God of Thunder, dressed as a bride to trick the King of the Giants, the groom, into returning his hammer. Hercules, a Roman god/man, posed as a female slave of Queen Lydia, who married him after he was exposed as a man. And who can forget Dustin Hoffman dressing as Dorothy in the movie *Tootsie*?

On the other side, Saint Margaret and Saint Joan of Arc disguised themselves as men in their pursuit of religious vocation. Diane Keaton in *Annie Hall* turned menswear into *the* hot trend in women's wear. What about Tilda Swinton going from male to female throughout time in *Orlando*?

Some suggestions:

- Go to the mall with him wearing her panties under his clothes and her in his jeans and a tight top or his shirt and tight jeans or leggings.

- Plan a night out with her in menswear.

- Dress him like a rocker from the androgynous '70s, and don't forget the makeup.

- Shave or wax his chest, legs, and pubic hair, and put him in silk PJs.

- Add a man's fedora to her strap-on and boots ensemble.

. . . .

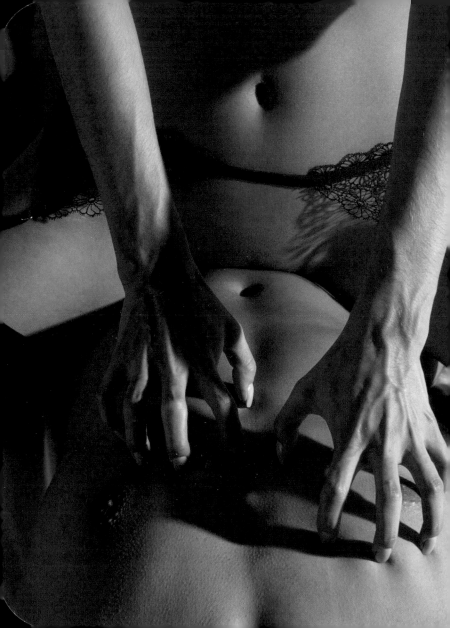

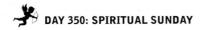 **DAY 350: SPIRITUAL SUNDAY**

Breaking Down the Pleasure Barriers

What keeps a woman from reaching orgasm? An active brain, according to studies underway at the University of Groningen in the Netherlands. Brain scans of women show that during high arousal, activity rose in one sensory part of the brain, but slowed down in the amygdala and hippocampus, areas that keep women tense during sex by, among other things, making to-do lists. The findings seem to confirm what other studies (not to mention conventional wisdom) have reported: Women need to be relaxed and free of distractions to enjoy sex. Men tune out distractions. And what can you do with a relaxed penis?

Still, researchers were surprised at the extraordinary deactivation in so many areas of the brain during orgasm. Only one tiny part was more active. The cerebellum coordinates movement and may also play a role in controlling emotions. Today create some relaxation rituals for her.

Some suggestions:

- Learn some techniques from meditation, such as deep breathing and mind clearing.

- Take a ten-minute break—no interactions.

- Do easy yoga poses.

- Learn Buddhist chants.

- Have a cup of tea or glass of wine at the same time each day to create a relaxing ritual.

....

DAY 351: FLIRTATION AND FOREPLAY MONDAY

Let Him See Your Book

Any time you can surprise your partner, you titillate him (or her). You do something that makes him look more closely at you and ask himself, "What is she thinking?" Completing one another's sentences may be comforting, but it isn't sexy.

Let him see the book you tuck into your tote bag. It should be something he would not expect you to be reading.

Some suggestions:

- *Sex Tips for Straight Women from a Gay Man*

- *Justine* (by the Marquis de Sade)

- *Size Matters: The Hard Facts About Male Sexuality That Every Woman Should Know*

- *The Best of Lesbian Erotica*

- *Masters of Sex*

- *Satyricon USA*

- *Diary of an Adulterous Woman*

....

The Come-from-Behind Hand Job Quickie

This story from a SexyPrime reader is very popular with men. He was staying in a hotel in Vegas, where he hooked up with an old lover. She told him to stand naked in front of a floor-to-ceiling window, and then gave him a memorable experience.

Then from behind, she caressed my cock and slowly stroked it. I put my hands up against the window glass from the pleasure.

With her other hand, she reached down between my legs and grasped my balls. She pulled them slightly back and kept playing with them while jacking me off with her left hand. As she worked the stroke, she pulled my cock lower, and that made it harder and harder.

When I was about to cum, she quickly aimed my cock at the window. Streams of cum shot down the glass. She continued stroking it as she moved her body around to the front. She put my cock into her mouth. Pumping in her mouth felt so good after that incredible orgasm.

....

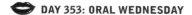 **DAY 353: ORAL WEDNESDAY**

No More Faking!

Surveys consistently show that 80 percent (and higher) of women fake orgasm, at least occasionally. Ladies, please. This has got to stop.

Faking reinforces his belief that his moves (that aren't working) are stellar. If he is your life partner, you have set up the classic disappointing sex scenario: She never comes and loses interest in sex but he keeps pestering her for it because he has no idea that she's never come. And if he is a casual lover, you just made it harder for another woman to be honest with him.

Declare today Unilateral Forgiveness of Orgasmic Debt Day. Don't hurt him by telling him how long and how often you've faked it. But do tell him what you want, what you need, and how to give it to you NOW. End the faking, and claim your pleasure!

....

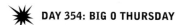 **DAY 354: BIG O THURSDAY**

Orgasm Control

Known as "edging," "peaking," "surfing," and several other less commonly used names, orgasm control is a collection of sexual techniques expressed in two ways. The active partner, or giver, controls the passive partner's orgasm, as in Orgasmic Providing (page 317). Or one person, usually the man, controls his own orgasm during masturbation or intercourse.

You have learned to use techniques for delaying male ejaculation, expanding and extending orgasm, and encouraging whole-body orgasm for men and women. The same skills set, especially the Venus Butterfly (page 31), is used in *The One-Hour Orgasm*, Leah and Bob Schwartz's 1995 best-seller, and is also the basis of extended massive orgasm.

The objective is to keep arousal high by varying the intensity and speed of stimulation, because the longer you remain in that highly aroused state, the more intense your orgasm will be. Many people who take the practice to the limits report feelings of euphoria. If you want to explore, try these sources:

- Sexy Spirits website, www.sexyspirits.com

- Research studies on orgasm control (and related names) conducted under scientific protocol. The archives of *The Journal of Sex Research* are a good place to start.

- Tantric and Taoist teachings. Margot Anand's *The Art of Sexual Ecstasy* is the best book ever written on the subject.

- Finally, if you read popular books such as *The One-Hour Orgasm*, recognize that the authors are teaching you the same skills you learned here, dressed up in hyper-hype and overpromising. Are you really going to have a one-hour orgasm?

. . . .

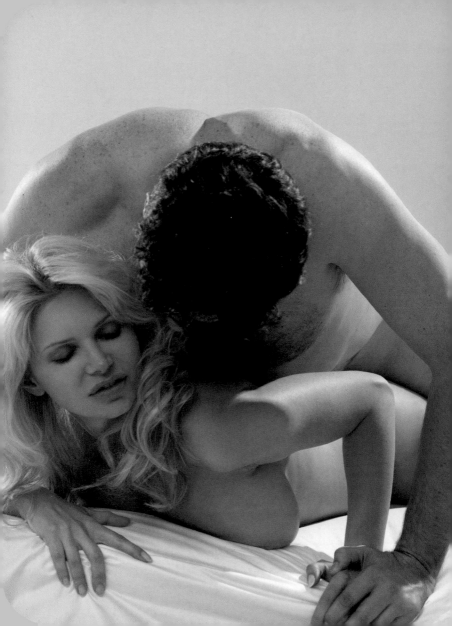

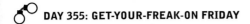

DAY 355: GET-YOUR-FREAK-ON FRIDAY

What Is Sexually "Normal"?

"Am I normal?" is one of the questions most often asked of sex experts. We all love sex surveys because they give us a group snapshot of sexual behaviors and show us just where we fit into this particular group. The sexual "normal" changes over time. A few generations ago, nice girls didn't suck cock. That is certainly not true anymore—especially for white women. (Sex behavior studies typically find that black, Hispanic, and Asian Americans are more sexually conservative than whites are.)

Here are some "normal" sex behavior statistics presented in the spirit of fun:

- Sex lasts three to ten minutes.

- The average couple has sex two or three times per week.

- He prefers rear entry; she, the missionary position.

- According to *The New England Journal of Medicine*, 68 percent of men and 59 percent of women have been involved with a person about whom their significant other does not know. (If you ask the readers of *Playboy*, the numbers are higher; the numbers are lower for readers of women's magazines.)

- Fifty percent of men have told a blatant lie (e.g., "I'm not married") to get sex.

- More than half of heterosexual couples have tried anal sex at least once.

. . . .

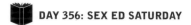 **DAY 356: SEX ED SATURDAY**

The Tantra Orgasm

Strictly speaking, the lovers are supposed to be in the Yab-Yum position (page 361) and the intense buildup to orgasm should last thirty minutes for us to label this an *official* Tantra orgasm. I borrowed a little from the traditionalist David Ramsdale, author of *Sexual Energy Ecstasy*, and the more pragmatic sexpert Lou Paget to create a Tantra orgasm for the rest of us.

In any intercourse position, she contracts her PC muscle around his penis while he remains still. No pelvic thrusting!

Caress and kiss and eye gaze while remaining motionless (except for the PC flexing) below the waist.

Hold this until the desire to thrust is unbearable. (Try to last at least ten minutes for a more intense orgasm.) The connection between the two of you should feel almost transcendent at this point.

Thrust as slowly as you can, until there is no denying the orgasms are ready to explode.

....

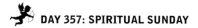 **DAY 357: SPIRITUAL SUNDAY**

Sacred Prostitute Day

The New Age Tantra gurus did not invent sacred sexuality. Unless you have studied the history of sex (or religions), you probably don't know that temple priestesses were sacred prostitutes in many cultures. Although the clergy fathered many illegitimate children, the Christian church turned sex into sin. Christians have not quite recovered from that. And look what the ayatollahs have done to Islam in the Middle East!

Have you heard of St. Aphra? The patron saint of reformed prostitutes, she was a sacred prostitute in the Temple of Venus and perhaps the Temple of Aphrodite. After her conversion, she was burned at the stake for being on the wrong side of church politics at the time. The stories of the Christian divine usually end badly in torment of one sort or another. Go online or to a bookstore and seek out some goddess/sacred prostitute role models today. Rituals typically include sexual dancing, fellatio, and intercourse with a highly talented vagina.

Some suggestions:

- Astarte, Phoenician goddess of love

- Ardan, Celtic goddess of love

- Branwen, Irish goddess of love

- Freya, German goddess of love

- Isis, Egyptian goddess of love

- Juno, Roman goddess of love

- Ursula, Haitian goddess of love

. . . .

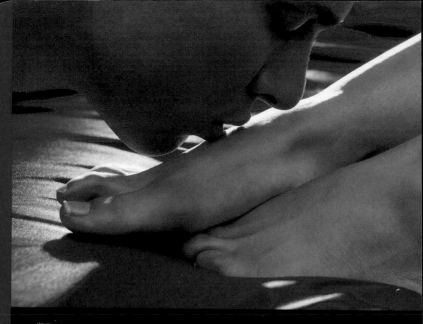

DAY 358: FLIRTATION AND FOREPLAY MONDAY

Play Footsies

It's an oldie but a goodie. Take your shoe off and rub your lover's foot with your foot. Then run your foot up and down her (his) leg.

Playing footsies while dining out or sitting in a movie theater is sexy, and it's a good game to play when you're side by side on the sofa, watching TV at the end of a long day. The foot is a sensuous appendage. Get those toes working.

....

The Good-Bye Quickie

She has an early flight. No time for sex, not even a quickie. But she looks so appealing, walking around the bedroom in her underwear, tossing items into her carry-on bag.

There *is* time. (Go back to the five-minute quickie on page 307.) You just need to persuade her of that—and fast.

Some suggestions:

- Put your hands on her forearms, look into her eyes, and say as seriously as you can, "You are so beautiful, I'll die if I don't have you right now."

- Barter—sex for completion of some onerous chore in her absence.

- Promises—chocolates, champagne, roses, or an erotic massage upon her return.

- The direct approach—put some lube on your fingers, grab her in your arms, and stroke her clit while you kiss her passionately.

Fifty-one weeks ago, you might have struck out with any or all of these approaches. Today, I am betting on you. (The more sex you have, the more sex you want.)

....

"69" with Hand Moves

Isn't simultaneously giving and receiving oral sex enough—without adding hand moves? Yes, but . . .

The hand moves allow you to sustain your partner's arousal when you have to take your mouth away because you're just too excited to have your teeth that close to your lover's genitals.

His Hand Moves

- Put two fingers in the shape of a V along the sides of her clitoris. When you pull your mouth away, gently press in with those fingers. Then move them up and down, stroking the sides.

- Keep one hand in the shape of a C around her clitoris. When you pull your mouth away, press in gently and then circle the hand, twisting your wrist.

- Keep two fingers inside her vagina, stimulating her G-spot, while you are performing cunnilingus and while taking a break.

Her Hand Moves

- Keep one hand around the base of his penis and move it up and down the shaft as needed, varying the speed depending on his arousal level, and faster when you take your mouth away.

- If his erection begins to wilt when you take your mouth away, put both hands around the shaft, fingers loosely woven together, and use upward strokes only on the shaft, rubbing your thumb across the frenulum and corona at the top of the upstroke.

- Cradle his balls in one hand, with your thumb ready to stroke his perineum.

....

 DAY 361: BIG O THURSDAY

Your Orgasm Story

We all have an orgasm story. For some women, the story is: *I can't come with him* or *I can't come at all.* For some men, the story is: *I come too fast.* Those may have been your stories a year ago. Or your stories may have been: *I wish I had more orgasms* or *I wish I had orgasms more easily.* Or maybe you wished for multiple orgasms, or, in his case, a shorter refractory period.

Our stories about ourselves—whether sex or money or family or others—are important because they influence how we behave, what we expect, and how we share ourselves with others, including our most intimate partners.

What's your orgasm story now?

Tell one another your story, or write it, if you are more comfortable reading than telling.

....

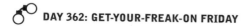

Second Life Sex

In the virtual world known as Second Life, real people spend real money to buy the play money that fuels their avatar's life. If you can peek into Second Life, it might be interesting. Here are some game rules:

- Seduction is text chat in graphic terms.

- Some participants move to Skype or the phone.

- They buy provocative outfits for their avatars or purchase "skins" to make them appear nude.

- Genitals must be purchased separately.

- More money must be spent on beds and accoutrements, such as vibrators and BDSM props.

- Nudity and sexual behavior are forbidden in Second Life outside of private areas and sex clubs.

....

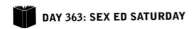
Plan a Sex Ed Curriculum

The Daily Sex Bible gives you many tantalizing tidbits of knowledge. I hope you will pursue subjects that particularly interest you in more depth and do searches for information that informs and expands your own sexuality.

Some categories to research:

- Sexual practices in the ancient world

- Erotic art, poetry, and literature

- The mythology of sex goddesses and gods and temple prostitutes

- Sacred sexuality

- Tantra

- New sex research

- Evolving trends in cybersex

- Sex tips from call girls and courtesans

- The practices of sexual adventurers, such as BDSM players, swingers, and people involved in polyamory

. . . .

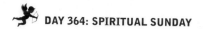 **DAY 364: SPIRITUAL SUNDAY**

The Sexual Thanksgiving

Make a puja (home worship) at your altars to the phallus and the vulva
(see pages 51 and 67). Arrange small bud vases of fresh blooms. Light
candles and incense. Put out little glasses of wine as offerings to the
gods and goddesses.

Now worship one another. Be thankful for a partner so erotically
creative as this one who has been game to try 365 days of new sex.
Share orgasms and be grateful.

Sexual gratitude is a powerful emotion, capable of transforming tense or
tired relationships.

....

"Have I told you lately that I *want* you?"

Women and men like to hear "I love you" and "I need you" and "You are beautiful (handsome)." But "I *want* you," said with quiet intensity, can trump any of those declarations on any given day.

To be desired sexually is to be fully realized as a woman or a man.

Let your partner know you desire her (him). Show her how much. Then start all over again with *The Daily Sex Bible*, this time picking and choosing your favorites from all the sex recipes in the book.

....

INDEX